Geriatric Medicine and Healthy Aging

Edited by Élvio Rúbio Gouveia,
Bruna Raquel Gouveia, Adilson Marques
and Andreas Ihle

Published in London, United Kingdom

Geriatric Medicine and Healthy Aging
http://dx.doi.org/10.5772/intechopen.98018
Edited by Élvio Rúbio Gouveia, Bruna Raquel Gouveia, Adilson Marques and Andreas Ihle

Contributors
Debanjan Banerjee, Abhishek Ramesh, Dabota Yvonne Buowari, Nafiseh Shokri-Mashhadi, Sharon Shiovitz-Ezra, Ohad Parag, Howard Litwin, Esmaeil Mehraeen, Ahmadreza Shamsabadi, Zahra Pashaei, Amy Joy Lanou, Tasha Woodall, Jeff Jones, Thomas Smythe, Louise Wooley Noble, Emma Olson, Lauren Alexa Gambrill, Élvio Rúbio Gouveia, Andreas Ihle, Adilson Marques, Bruna R. Gouveia, Priscila Marconcin

First published in London, United Kingdom, 2023 by IntechOpen
IntechOpen is the global imprint of INTECHOPEN LIMITED, registered in England and Wales, registration number: 11086078, 5 Princes Gate Court, London, SW7 2QJ, United Kingdom

British Library Cataloguing-in-Publication Data
A catalogue record for this book is available from the British Library

Additional hard and PDF copies can be obtained from orders@intechopen.com

Geriatric Medicine and Healthy Aging
Edited by Élvio Rúbio Gouveia, Bruna Raquel Gouveia, Adilson Marques and Andreas Ihle
p. cm.
Print ISBN 978-1-80355-828-8
Online ISBN 978-1-80355-829-5
eBook (PDF) ISBN 978-1-80355-830-1

Meet the editors

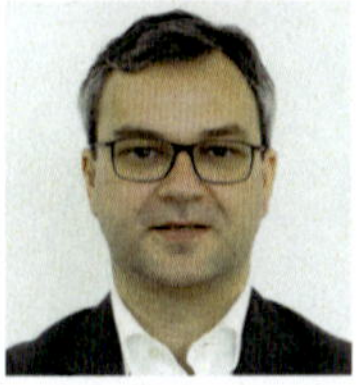

Élvio Rúbio Gouveia (ERG) has a degree in Physical Education, a Master in Physical Education, and a PhD in Sport Sciences. ERG is an Assistant Professor at the University of Madeira and Vice President of the Interactive Technologies Institute, a research unit from the Laboratory of Robotics and Engineering Systems. ERG also collaborates with the Center for the Interdisciplinary Study of Gerontology and Vulnerability, University of Geneva. ERG has been developing and evaluating strategies to promote physical activity, fitness, and quality of life. Focusing on the physiological assessment of human fitness and the promotion of healthy ageing, his research is grounded on a multidisciplinary approach to several issues that affect healthy fitness.

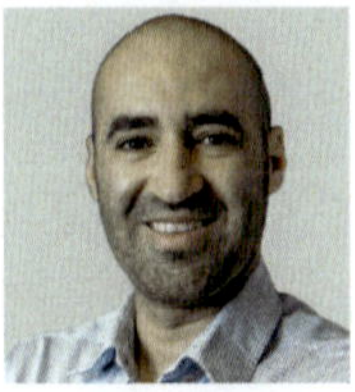

Adilson Marques is a professor at the University of Lisbon. He was a physical education teacher for several years and a coach in scholar sports programs. His main research interest is the study of health promotion and physical activity, and mental health. He has published several international peer-reviewed original articles and has been an investigator in several research projects. He is a reviewer for several scientific journals in sports science and health promotion. For six years, he was a Portuguese Society of Physical Education board member. He is a team member of the National Physical Activity Promotion Program at the Portuguese Ministry of Health.

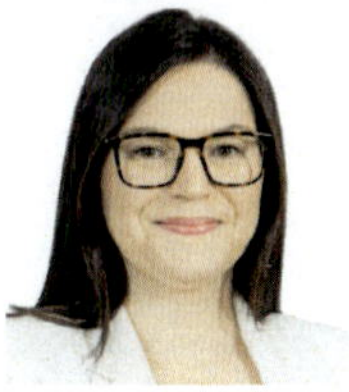

Bruna Raquel Gouveia (BRG) is an Adjunct Professor at the Saint Joseph of Cluny Higher School of Nursing, where she coordinates the Master's Program in Rehabilitation Nursing. She is a researcher at ITI – LARSyS and CIGEV - Geneva University, and a full European Academy of Nursing Sciences member. She has been the Deputy Director of Health of the Autonomous Region of Madeira since 2020. She coordinates the Department of Strategic Planning and Global Health, supporting the design, coordination, and implementation of the region's health politics. Her research has focused on studying human development and aging and the evaluation of complex interventions in rehabilitation and health. Currently, BRG is working in epidemiological research and developing and using innovative technologies for health. One example is the use of smart information systems for the epidemiological surveillance of COVID-19 in Madeira.

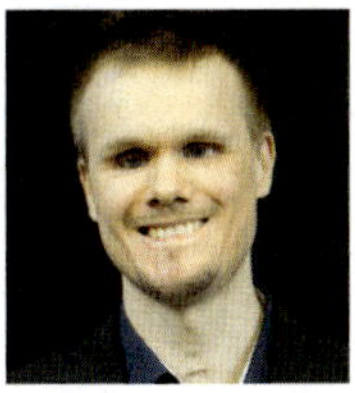

Andreas Ihle is a professor at the University of Geneva, Switzerland. He received his MSc in Psychology from the University of Dresden, Germany, and his PhD in Psychology from the University of Geneva. His interdisciplinary research focuses on better understanding human development across the lifespan, such as explaining the enormous inter- and intraindividual differences in cognitive functioning, health, well-being, activity engagement, reserve accumulation, and vulnerabilities from early childhood to late adulthood. On these topics, he has published several international peer-reviewed journal articles. He is a reviewer for a broad variety of scientific journals and funding agencies.

Contents

Preface

Living a long and healthy life is now considered the main challenge of societies worldwide. The World Health Organization (WHO) in 2015 defined healthy aging as the "ongoing process of developing and maintaining the functional ability that enables well-being in older age." Functional ability is a central concept in this approach since it comprises the interaction between physical and mental capacities in a particular environment. Physical activity has been considered a key recommendation for developing sustainable policies and action programs for healthy aging. Increasing physical activity is a necessary condition to maintain functional and cognitive abilities as well as social activities. Currently, assisted living technologies have been given special attention since innovative information and communication technology (ICT)-based products can make a real difference in people's physical, mental, and social lives. Considering the multifaceted character of the phenomenon, all these predictors directly impact health-related quality of life.

Geriatric Medicine and Healthy Aging is organized into four sections and eight chapters. Section 1, "Healthy Aging: An Overview", includes an introductory chapter that introduces and defines the main concepts of this book: healthy aging, physical activity, functional fitness, cognitive function, and assisted living technologies. The chapter explains how each independent variable can explain the variance in quality of life in older people and considers the relationship between these concepts. The chapter also identifies priorities, challenges, and future research with the purpose of creating solutions in health and well-being adapted to the needs of older people.

Chapter 2, "Exercise Aging and Health: A Proposal Course for Healthcare Professionals and Physical Activity Instructors", proposes a curriculum to be taught to healthcare professionals, physical activity instructors, or other health professionals who work directly with older people. The curriculum addresses structural topics, including aspects of aging (i.e., demography, theories, and current policies on aging) and physical and functional aged-related declines, including morphological and physiological changes. Physical–psychosocial relationships are also explored, focusing on the relationships between aging, active life, cognitive function, physical activity, well-being, and health-related quality of life. Finally, the chapter presents guidelines for exercise prescription in the older population, including general guidelines for pre-exercise assessment and critical considerations for maximizing the effective development of exercise programs for older people. This curriculum is expected to support professionals with theoretical knowledge regarding exercise, aging, and health in different contexts of intervention with older people (i.e., health gyms, rehabilitation centers, elderly centers, city councils, and parish councils, among others). This course content is believed to be an essential step in improving the quality of physical activity programs for older people.

Chapter 3, "Perspective Chapter: Geriatric Care in Africa", explores the issue of geriatric care on the African continent. It presents emerging needs, identifying the most vulnerable groups and Africa's shortage of qualified geriatricians. This chapter underlines Africa's health and social problems and emphasizes several challenges that make older people prone to vulnerabilities. Another enormous problem presented is the lack of technical training for geriatricians. The conclusion is that there are few geriatricians in Africa and thus it is essential to consider partnerships between African counties and other more developed countries to find strategies for training in geriatric medicine, such as postgraduate courses, fellowships, refresher courses, and workshops.

Section 2, "Physical–psychosocial Relationships: Moving towards Healthy Aging", explores physical–psychosocial relationships and how they affect healthy aging.

Chapter 4, "Does Physical Activity Mediate the Effect of Loneliness on Inflammatory and Metabolic Processes?", clarifies the contribution of physical activity to the associations between loneliness and immune and metabolic processes and provides insights concerning the mechanism by which this social–biological connection operates. This chapter supports the idea that loneliness is associated with increased levels of inflammation. It also suggests that loneliness is associated with subsequent low metabolic regulation, as manifested by elevated concentrations in all three metabolic measures of body mass index (BMI), hemoglobin A1C (Hba1c), and serum cystatin C (CysC). In conclusion, this chapter observes an important psycho-physiological mechanism that may be present among older adults. A strong public health message to engage in physical activities in late life also mitigates the deleterious health effects of loneliness.

Directly connected with the topic of physical–psychosocial relationships, Chapter 5, "Perspective Chapter: Social Distancing and Isolation – Unintended Consequences, Concerns, and Antidotes for Older Adults", explores the consequences of social isolation, particularly in the post–COVID-19 pandemic period. This chapter stresses that opportunities for increasing the social connectedness of older adults and others who are isolated must be prioritized to decrease the impact of social isolation and loneliness on mental and physical health. In addition, it proposes recommendations for policies, programs, and other actions addressing social isolation as a determinant of healthy aging using case examples from the western region of North Carolina.

Section 3, "Novel Approaches to Prevention and Treatment of Age-Related Declines", addresses novel approaches to the prevention and treatment of age-related declines.

Chapter 6, "Perspective Chapter: The Role of Modifiable Factors, Particularly Nutritional Factors, on Age-Related Sarcopenia", explores nutrition as a modifiable factor in fighting against sarcopenia and frailty. Sarcopenia, which is defined by low muscle strength, low muscle mass, and low physical performance, has been highly correlated with poor quality of life, risk of falls, fractures, and higher healthcare costs. Despite the growing interest in treating this phenomenon, the lack of adequate knowledge underlying the multi-factorial parthenogenesis of age-sarcopenia hinders the diagnosis of effective therapeutic approaches. This chapter discusses the association between the components of sarcopenia and nutritional status in older adults and their potential effect on prevention and treatment.

Chapter 7, "Perspective Chapter: Nutraceuticals as a Therapeutic Promise in Healthy Aging and Neurocognitive Disorders", explores modern therapeutics, namely, approaches based on chemical substances belonging to classes of natural dietary origin that seem to have protective properties against some age-related diseases, including neurodegenerative ones.

Section 4, "Assisted Living: Technology for Healthy Aging", includes Chapter 8, "Perspective Chapter: Telehealth Technologies for the Elderly People", which presents a systematic review of the literature on telemedicine tools for older adults from a perspective of empowering them to take an active role in the management of their health. The chapter also emphasizes the need for co-creation and co-design with end users to ensure adequate technological solutions.

Élvio Rúbio Gouveia
Department of Physical Education and Sport,
University of Madeira,
Madeira, Portugal

Laboratory of Robotics and Systems in Engineering and Science (LARSyS),
Interactive Technologies Institute,
Funchal, Portugal

Center for the Interdisciplinary Study of Gerontology and Vulnerability,
University of Geneva,
Geneva, Switzerland

Adilson Marques
Interdisciplinary Centre for the Study of Human Performance (CIPER),
Faculty of Human Kinetics,
University of Lisbon,
Lisbon, Portugal

Instituto de Saúde Ambiental (ISAMB),
University of Lisbon,
Lisbon, Portugal

Bruna Raquel Gouveia
Center for the Interdisciplinary Study of Gerontology and Vulnerability,
University of Geneva,
Geneva, Switzerland

Regional Directorate of Health,
Secretary of Health of the Autonomous Region of Madeira,
Madeira, Portugal

Saint Joseph of Cluny Higher School of Nursing,
Funchal, Portugal

Andreas Ihle
Center for the Interdisciplinary Study of Gerontology and Vulnerability,
University of Geneva,
Geneva, Switzerland

Department of Psychology,
University of Geneva,
Geneva, Switzerland

Swiss National Centre of Competence in Research
LIVES—Overcoming Vulnerability, Life Course Perspectives,
Switzerland

Section 1

Healthy Aging: An Overview

Chapter 1

Introductory Chapter: Healthy Aging, Physical Activity, Functional Fitness, Cognitive Function, and Assisted Living Technologies – The Ground for the Sustainability of Health and Quality of Life in Older People

Élvio Rúbio Gouveia, Bruna R. Gouveia, Adilson Marques and Andreas Ihle

1. Introduction

1.1 Sociodemographic change

Living a long and healthy life is considered the main challenge of societies worldwide. Accompanying a worldwide sociodemographic change, statistical data show an increase in the life expectancy of the most aged segment of the population [1]. Indeed, due to low birth rates, advancements in medical and pharmaceutical technology, health care, nutrition, and sanitation have resulted in lower death rates worldwide [2]. People are living longer, and the population worldwide is growing older. The current increase in the number of older people, combined with the increase in chronic diseases and disabilities associated with age (including limitations in functional fitness components, often due to falls and physical and cognitive alterations, predictors of immobility and dementia), present our societies with global social, economic, and health challenges.

1.2 Healthy aging

The WHO [3] defined healthy aging as the "ongoing process of developing and maintaining the functional ability that enables wellbeing in older age." Functional ability is a central concept in this approach since it comprises the interaction between physical and mental capacities in a particular environment. Nowadays, it is imperative to develop effective healthy aging strategies because, as previously mentioned, most people expect to live beyond 60 years. By 2050, 1 in 5 people will be 60 or older [1]. This means that more and more people live longer, which poses new challenges and opportunities to the community. However, there seems to be no doubt that a person's general health is a significant factor to consider among successful aging strategies so that people can benefit from the extra years of life they have achieved, doing what they value.

1.3 Physical activity and functional fitness relationships

Evidence supports that an active and independent lifestyle in old age fundamentally depends on a person's functional fitness levels, for which balance and cognition are significant [4, 5]. Physical activity (PA) has been considered a key recommendation for developing sustainable policies and action programs for healthy aging. Increasing PA is necessary to maintain functional and cognitive abilities and social activities [4, 6].

Currently, a body of evidence has reported many health and performance-related benefits of engaging in regular PA. It has been shown that certain levels of functional fitness protect the individual from many chronic diseases, promote better performances in daily living activities, and enhance participation in various sports and recreational activities [2, 7]. Strategies to promote PA and functional fitness have been considered priorities for many organizations with worldwide expressions, such as ACSM, WHO, and the Centers for Disease Control and Prevention (CDC). These organizations have developed powerful campaigns centred on promoting exercise and regular physical activity as a means for older people to become healthier, maintain an independent lifestyle, and improve their quality of life and functional capacity.

Research efforts support that the association between PA and functional fitness is reciprocal; functional fitness provides the individual with the capability to engage in physical activities, whereas PA helps to maintain and, in some cases, improve functional fitness [4, 8, 9]. The health and performance-related benefits of regular participation in PA, particularly in older people, are well documented [9, 10]. People who manage to maintain a certain level of functional fitness gain some protection concerning various health conditions (e.g., heart disease, diabetes, obesity, cancers), as well as being able to guarantee the execution of activities of daily living in an independent and safe [11–13]. Additionally, benefits at the psychological level are also evident, especially concerning emotional well-being, increased cognitive function, and a high perception of quality of life [14].

Although this dose-response relationship between increased levels of PA and the onset of chronic diseases or functional disabilities is relatively well documented [15–17], only a small percentage of older people engage in regular physical activity. Older people continue to spend more time in sedentary activities (i.e., time sitting), directly affecting many physiological systems, such as cardiorespiratory and musculoskeletal health [18, 19]. Reference literature on the epidemiology of physical activity has reinforced the direct relationship between the increase in sedentary activity associated with morpho-functional limitations related to age and the onset of chronic diseases or disabilities [19]. This is a crucial subject because it is directly related to the loss of autonomy, reduced quality of life, and increased social support and health care costs.

1.4 Assisted living technologies

Assisted living technologies have been given special attention since innovative ICT-based products can make a real difference in people's physical, mental, and social lives. According to the World Health Organization, in 2019, the following diseases were among the top 10 causes of death in the world: (1) Ischaemic heart disease; (2) stroke; (3) chronic obstructive pulmonary disease; (4) lower respiratory infections; (5) trachea, bronchus, lung cancers; (6) Alzheimer's disease and other dementias; and (7) Diabetes mellitus. These causes of death have several common denominators, including frailty, physical immobility, and various risk factors associated with cardiovascular, metabolic, respiratory, and cognitive function. Practical actions and making the most of technologies to reverse these problems are priorities. In this context, many health organizations have tried to combat these problems through various disease prevention and control actions (i.e., educational actions, screenings, and wearable health devices) to delay their appearance or lessen their severity. This allows older people to remain a valuable resource in their families, communities, and economies while maintaining high levels of independence and quality of life. Additionally, and no less importantly, this proactive approach reduces the need for institutionalization and significantly contributes to the sustainability of Health Systems. It has been identified as a strategic priority to increase health and social responses to problems arising from demographic aging (such as frequent and prolonged hospitalizations and difficulties in reintegrating into the community after hospital discharge). Assisted living technologies focused on applications in the health area could significantly reduce the number of older people who overuse emergency health services.

Faced with this reality, which is a problem that cuts across many communities around the world, among strategies for the prevention and control of health signs, great attention and investment has been given to the development of Wearable Health Devices, with the function of assisting people in monitoring their health status, providing data with potential for diagnosis and early referral of treatment [20]. Some so-called developed countries have increasingly invested in developing this innovative monitoring system, integrating sensors capable of monitoring deficits and functional mobility, cardiovascular disease, metabolic disease, respiratory disease, and cognitive function, among others. It is for this reason that the revenue of the world wearable health devices market has already reached around 26 billion US dollars, with expectations of reaching 34 billion dollars still in 2019 [21].

Although there is great hope for the potential positive effects of using this type of Assisted Technologies in the monitoring and support of health care, which includes the integration of multimodal signal processing systems for the quantification and evaluation of human activity, physiological, behavioral, emotional and cognitive with real-time feedback, scientific evidence on the validation and effectiveness of the use of these devices is still insufficient for several reasons [20]. Firstly, there still needs to be a consensus regarding the evaluation parameters to be integrated into the monitoring systems and the validation of data collected for diagnosis and early referral in the therapeutic plan. Secondly, only a few wearable health devices have been concerned with integrating information from the user's interaction with the system, losing an essential source of information in the psychosocial area. Thirdly, most systems available on the market operate in isolation (i.e., in a disintegrated and modular way), and the associated costs are still high for the end user. Finally, fourth place, and not least, it is necessary to break down barriers and resistance to using assisted technology in people's daily lives. To this end, the extra concern is needed in developing more adapted and 'friendly' interfaces for the elderly.

1.5 Final considerations

Considering the multifaceted character of the phenomenon, all these predictors directly impact health-related quality of life. We identified priorities and challenges, boosting research, technological development, and innovation to create solutions in health and well-being adapted to the needs of older people. The future involves research, improving knowledge, and developing therapeutic resources centred on functional skills (mobility and cognitive performance) with positive implications for healthy aging.

Author details

Élvio Rúbio Gouveia[1,2,3]*, Bruna R. Gouveia[2,3,4,5], Adilson Marques[6,7]
and Andreas Ihle[3,8,9]

1 Department of Physical Education and Sport, University of Madeira, Portugal

2 Laboratory of Robotics and Systems in Engineering and Science (LARSyS), Interactive Technologies Institute, Portugal

3 Center for the Interdisciplinary Study of Gerontology and Vulnerability, University of Geneva, Switzerland

4 Saint Joseph of Cluny Higher School of Nursing, Portugal

5 Regional Health Directorate, Secretary of Health and Civil Protection of the Autonomous Region of Madeira, Portugal

6 Interdisciplinary Centre for the Study of Human Performance (CIPER), Faculty of Human Kinetics, University of Lisbon, Portugal

7 Instituto de Saúde Ambiental (ISAMB), University of Lisbon, Portugal

8 Department of Psychology, University of Geneva, Switzerland

9 Swiss National Centre of Competence in Research LIVES—Overcoming Vulnerability: Life Course Perspectives, Switzerland

*Address all correspondence to: erubiog@staff.uma.pt

References

[1] European Commission. European Commission Report on the Impact of Demographic Change. 2020. Available from: https://commission.europa.eu/system/files/2020-06/demography_report_2020_n.pdf

[2] Jones CJ, Rose DJ. Physical Activity Instruction of Older Adults. Champaign, IL: Human Kinetics; 2005

[3] World Health Organization. World Report on Ageing and Health. Geneva: World Health Organization; 2015. Available from: https://apps.who.int/iris/handle/10665/186463

[4] Gouveia ER, Maia JA, Beunen GP, Blimkie CR, Fena E, Freitas DL. Functional fitness and physical activity of Portuguese community-residing older adults. Journal of Aging and Physical Activity. 2013;**21**(1):1-19

[5] Ihle A, Ghisletta P, Gouveia ÉR, Gouveia BR, Oris M, Maurer J, et al. Lower executive functioning predicts steeper subsequent decline in well-being only in young-old but not old-old age. International Journal of Behavioral Development. 2021;**45**(2):97-108

[6] Gouveia ER, Ihle A, Gouveia BR, Kliegel M, Marques A, Freitas DL. Muscle mass and muscle strength relationships to balance: The role of age and physical activity. Journal of Aging and Physical Activity. 2019;**4**:1-7. DOI: 10.1123/japa.2018-0113

[7] Rikli RE, Jones CJ. Senior Fitness Test Manual. Champaign, IL: Human Kinetics; 2013

[8] Rimmer JH. Assessment issues related to physical activity and disability. In: Zhu W, Chodzko-Zajko W, editors. Measurement Issues in Aging and Physical Activity. Proceedings of the 10th Measurement and Evaluation Symposium. Champaign, IL: Human Kinetics; 2006. pp. 69-79

[9] Shepard RJ. Aerobic Fitness and Health. Champaign, IL: Human Kinetics; 1994

[10] Bouchard C, Shephard RJ. Physical activity, fitness, and health: The model and key concepts. In: Bouchard C, Shephard RJ, Stephens T, editors. Physical Activity, Fitness, and Health: International Proceedings and Consensus Statement. Champaign IL: Human kinetics; 1994. pp. 77-88

[11] He XZ, Baker DW. Body mass index, physical activity, and the risk of decline in overall health and physical functioning in late middle age. American Journal of Public Health. 2004;**94**:1567-1573

[12] Hillsdon MM, Brunner EJ, Guralnik JM, Marmot MG. Prospective study of physical activity and physical function in early old age. The American Journal of Preventive Medicine. 2005;**28**:245-250

[13] Leveille SG, Guralnik JM, Ferrucci L, Langlois JA. Aging successfully until death in old age: Opportunities for increasing active life expectancy. American Journal of Epidemiology. 1999;**149**:654-664

[14] Ihle A, Gouveia ER, Gouveia BR, Orsholits D, Kliegel M. Ageing and Reserves. In: Dario S, Eric W, editors. Withstanding Vulnerability throughout Adult Life – Dynamics of Stressors, Resources, and Reserves. Singapore: Palgrave Macmillan, Springer Nature; 2023. pp. 239-252

[15] Kampert JB, Blair SN, Barlow CE, Kohl HW. Physical activity, physical fitness, and all-cause and cancer mortality: A prospective study of men and women. Annals of Epidemiology. 1996;**6**(5):452-457

[16] Kushi LH, Fee RM, Folsom AR, Mink PJ, Anderson KE, Sellers TA. Physical activity and mortality in postmenopausal women. The Journal of the American Medical Association. 1997;**277**(16):1287-1292

[17] Paffenbarger RS, Hyde RT, Wing AL, Lee IM, Jung DL, Kampert JB. The association of changes in physical-activity level and other lifestyle characteristics with mortality among men. The New England Journal of Medicine. 1993;**328**(8):538-545

[18] American College of Sports Medicine. ACSM's Guidelines for Exercise Testing and Prescription. Eleventh ed. Philadelphia: Lippincott Williams & Wilkins; 2022

[19] Dishman RK, Heath GW, Min LI. Physical Activity Epidemiology (2° Education). Champaign, IL: Human Kinetics; 2013

[20] Dias D, Cunha JP. Wearable health devices-vital sign monitoring, systems and technologies. Sensors (Basel). 2018;**18**(8):2414. DOI: 10.3390/s18082414

[21] Statista BI. Wearable Device Sales Revenue Worldwide from 2016 to 2022 (in Billion U.S.Dollars). New York, NY, USA: Statista Inc.; 2017

Chapter 2

Exercise Aging and Health: A Proposal Course for Healthcare Professionals and Physical Activity Instructors

Élvio Rúbio Gouveia, Bruna R. Gouveia, Adilson Marques, Priscila Marconcin and Andreas Ihle

Abstract

To live a long and healthy life is now considered the main challenge of geriatric medicine worldwide. Exercise, aging, and health are key research topics to maintain functional ability that has been considered one of the strongest predictors of independence in old age. Functional ability comprises the interaction between physical and mental capacities in a particular environment. Increasing physical activity is considered a key recommendation in sustainable policies and action programs for healthy aging. Evidence shows that physical activity impacts functional and cognitive abilities and social activities. The contents of training courses related to Exercise Aging and Health are responsible for ensuring an intervention focused on the needs of older people. Healthcare professionals, physical activity instructors, or other health professionals who work directly with older people may need to understand deeply demography, theories, and current policies on aging, physical, and functional changes associated with aging, physical-psychosocial relationships, contextual determinants of physical activity, and exercise prescription in the older population.

Keywords: aging, exercise, functional ability, health, physical activity, training

1. Introduction

This chapter aims to present a content course proposal on the topic of "Exercise Aging and Health," to be taught to healthcare professionals, physical activity instructors, or other health professionals who work directly with older people. In a nutshell, the contents to be addressed include five main topics. The first topic addresses an introduction to the aspects of aging, including issues related to demography, theories, and current policies on aging. The second topic explores the physical and functional changes associated with aging. Morphological changes and physiological systems, i.e. body composition, cardiopulmonary, musculoskeletal, and nervous and sensory systems, are broadly described. Also, in this topic, functional changes are addressed, i.e. functional fitness and mobility. Topic 3 presents research on physical-psychosocial relationships, exploring the relationships between aging, active life, cognitive function, physical activity, well-being, and health-related quality of life. Topic 4 is dedicated to studying the contextual determinants of physical activity in the elderly. Here, the models of adoption and maintenance of physically active lifestyles are explored, as well as the Age-friendly Environments. Finally, the last topic is dedicated to the study of guidelines for exercise prescription in the older population. Here, general guidelines for pre-exercise assessment are outlined, as well as key considerations for maximizing the effective development of exercise programs for older people.

It is expected that students who take this course should be able to properly use theoretical knowledge regarding exercise, aging, and health in different contexts of intervention with older people (i.e. health gyms, rehabilitation centers, elderly centers, city councils, parish councils, among others). They should be able to adopt a scientific attitude and a critical reflective method in the face of research results from the assessment of the physical dimensions (morphological and functional) of the older person. They must show the capacity for initiative, innovation, and acceptable use of information regarding protocols and techniques for assessing functional fitness and know-how to assess the scientificity of the information collected on the relationships and interrelationships of physical activity and chronic diseases, as well as the benefits and risks associated with the regular practice of physical activity and/or exercise. They must systematically carry out a functional assessment of the older person, guaranteeing all safety conditions in the evaluation and intervention, as well as adequately interpreting the objective and subjective data of the physical dimensions assessment process, using this information to prescribe the exercise. Finally, they must be able to conceptualize an exercise plan adapted to a previously outlined functional profile.

2. Topic 1: introductory aspects of aging

2.1 Demography of aging

The demographic transition characterized by an aging population is a global phenomenon that directly impacts different sectors of society. The advancements in medical and pharmaceutical technology, nutrition, and sanitation have resulted in lower healthcare death worldwide. People are living longer, and the population worldwide is growing older. Recent key facts shown by the World Health Organization [1] underlines that between 2015 and 2050, the proportion of the population over 60 years will nearly double from 12 to 22%. Besides the mortality associated with COVID-19, people aged 60 years and older will outnumber children younger than 5 years by 2020. In the same document, it is written that all countries face significant challenges to ensure that their health and social systems are ready to deal with this demographic shift.

Cognitive, physical, and social stimulation can play a crucial role in delaying disability and maintaining the quality of life, allowing people to continue to do what they want, without pain and autonomously, for as long as possible. Additionally, age-related declines in cognitive, physical, and social function are an inevitable human condition that often results in socioeconomic and service overload. These age-associated changes increase the vulnerability of older people to chronic illness and mortality.

2.2 Concepts and theories of aging

Aging refers to a process or group of processes occurring in living organisms that, over time, lead to a loss of adaptability, functional impairments, and eventually death [2]. Taylor and Johnson [3] defined biological aging as slow, progressive, structural, and functional changes at the cellular, tissue, and organ levels, ultimately affecting the function of all body systems.

Numerous theories have been proposed to explain the process of aging but neither appears to be entirely satisfactory [4]. Taylor and Johnson [3] suggested that these can be grouped into five broad categories of aging: (i) wear and tear theories; (ii) genetics theories; (iii) general imbalance theories; (iv) accumulation theories; and (v) the dysdifferentiative hypothesis of aging and cancer.

Jones [5] divided the theories of aging into three main categories: biological, psychological, and sociological. Biological theories of aging—including genetic damage and gradual imbalance theories—focus on the factors that cause senescence of the body and increase the risk of morbidity and mortality with age. Psychological theories focus on the influence of psychological processes and personality characteristics on aging. Sociological theories focus on the impact of the social and physical environments on aging.

The modern biological theories of aging in humans fall into two main categories: programmed theories and damage or error theories [6]. The programmed theories imply that aging follows a biological timetable, perhaps a continuation of the one that regulates childhood growth and development. This regulation would depend on changes in gene expression that affect the systems responsible for maintenance, repair, and defense responses. The programmed theory has three subcategories: programmed longevity, endocrine theory, and immunological theory. The damage or error theories emphasize environmental assaults on living organisms that induce cumulative damage at various levels as the cause of aging. The damage or error theory includes wear and tear theory, rate of living theory, cross-linking free radical theory, and somatic DNA damage theory.

The complexity of aging derives from an aggregate of causes that led to the development and polarization of the theories of aging. In this context, Jones [5] and Jin [6] believe that no single theory thoroughly explains the phenomenon of the aging process, but each offers some clues. Many of the proposed theories interact with each other in a complex way.

2.3 Policies on aging

As previously mentioned, the WHO emphasizes the longevity achieved by the population, reinforcing that most people expect to live beyond 60 years. It is likely that by 2050 one in five people will be 60 years old or more [1]. This means that a longer life brings great opportunities. However, how each individual can benefit from the extra years depends largely on one key factor: *Health*. On the other hand, evidence suggests that older people do not have a better health status than earlier generations. Additionally, those who have experienced lifelong events have a higher risk of health problems.

In this context, the concept of “healthy aging” emerges, which is the focus of the WHO’s work on aging for 2015–2030. “Healthy aging” is understood as a process of developing and maintaining the functional capacity that enables the well-being of the elderly adult. This central concept emphasizes, on the one hand, the need for action focused on multiple sectors and, on the other hand, the possibility of older people continuing to be a valid resource in their families, communities, and economies. We understand that one of the most important messages that can be drawn from this WHO theory of healthy aging is that one of the main focuses of the work of gerontologists, and all professionals responsible for offering services to the elderly is to find strategies and concerted actions that help the older people to continue doing the things they value most for as long as possible [7]. Within the scope of policies for healthy aging, the WHO assumed five strategic goals: (1) commitment to action, that is, to establish models, strengthen the capacity to formulate evidence-based policies, and combat stigma and stereotype of aging; (2) aligning health systems with the needs of older adults, i.e. orienting health systems around individual needs and potential for involvement, ensuring accessibility to quality care, and ensuring the sustainability of healthcare; (3) develop age-friendly environments, through the promotion of autonomy, the involvement of older people, and the promotion of multisectoral actions; (4) strengthen long-term care, with a view to continuously improving a sustainable and equitable policy in terms of long-term care, also integrating caregivers; and (5) improve evaluation, monitoring, and research, defining the suitable instruments, methodologies, and protocols, strengthening research capacity and encouraging innovation, and sustaining evidence of the benefits of actions focused on healthy aging for the population.

As a continuing of the concept of healthy aging, in 2015 the WHO emphasized the concept of active aging, as a multidimension that involves physical functionality, urban environment, and social inclusion. The WHO defined active aging as "...the process of optimizing opportunities for health, participation, and security in order to enhance quality of life as people age" [7]. The concept of Active and Healthy Aging (AHA) comprehends the results of the interaction between the physical and mental capacity of an individual and the context of each individual's life.

3. Topic 2: physical and functional changes associated with aging

3.1 Morphological changes and physiological systems: Body composition and systems: Cardiopulmonary, musculoskeletal, nervous, and sensory

Although it is difficult to distinguish the effects of aging on the physiologic function of the impact of deconditioning or disease, the aging process leads to profound changes in the cardiopulmonary, musculoskeletal, nervous, and immune systems. For example, the American College of Sports Medicine (2018) states that the incidence of stroke decreases about 30% from 25 to 85 years of age; there is a progressive reduction of ventilatory peak flow and lung capacity with advancing age; there is an increased bone loss resulting in reduced bone mineral density; about 25% of muscle function, defined as the highest lifetime force-generating capacity, is lost by around 65 years of age. Also, negative changes of the central nervous system are observed in neurotransmitters, nerve conduction, and fine functional-fitness control.

Regarding the body composition and musculoskeletal changes, one of the major age effects of body composition faced by older people is a gradual loss of skeletal muscle mass and strength that occurs with advancing age, called Sarcopenia. Sarcopenia increases the risk of falls [8], is associated with cardiac disease and respiratory disease [9, 10], and increased risk of death [11, 12]. In addition, it is accompanied by functional decline and disability [13, 14]. With increasing age and from about

40–45 years old, lean soft tissue and skeletal muscle mass progressively decline [15]. Evidence shows that about 25% of muscle function, defined as the highest lifetime force-generating capacity, is lost by around 65 years of age [3].

Finally, it has been reported that cognitive functioning declines with age [2]. Cognitive function is the intellectual process by which a person becomes aware of ideas, perceives, and understands them. It involves all aspects of perception, thinking, remembering, learning, attention, vigilance, reasoning, and problem-solving. This concept includes psychomotor functioning (reaction time, movement time, and performance speed) [16]. There is evidence that regular physical exercise [17–19] and cognitive training [20, 21] are non-pharmaceutical interventions that attenuate age-related cognitive decline and improve cognitive performance in older people.

According to Fernández-Ballesteros [22], active daily cognitive activity and social and leisure activities have a positive impact on the general functioning of cognitive abilities. Therefore, social contacts and good integration of people in the community are factors that contribute to greater protection of cognitive functioning. In addition, there is some literature to support that interventions based on cognitive stimulation programs associated with group physical activity programs have great potential in older people with identified dementia and healthy older people [2, 3].

3.2 Functional changes: functional fitness and mobility

Among older adults, functional fitness is defined as the ability to perform activities of daily living normally, safely, independently, and without fatigue [23]. Improving functional fitness in older adults (i.e. lower and upper limb muscle strength, aerobic capacity, flexibility, and dynamic balance) is a critical factor in maintaining their independence in daily living activities. In this sense, a reduction in functional fitness levels is generally associated with a decline in general functional capacity and basic activities of daily living such as climbing stairs, walking, carrying groceries, and many other common tasks [3, 23]. Normative functional fitness scores have been published for older adults in different countries: United States of America [24]; Portugal [25]; Brazil [26]; Poland [27]; and China [28]. Results revealed a pattern of decline across most age groups on all variables. The total decrease in muscular strength, cardiorespiratory endurance, and agility/balance was about 30–45% between 60 and 94 years of age. The pattern of decrease over age was similar in men and women. However, men scored better on muscular strength, aerobic endurance, and agility/balance, and women scored better on flexibility [24–28].

4. Topic 3: physical-psychosocial relationships

4.1 Aging, active life, and cognitive function

Owing to the inevitable well-documented age-related losses in cognitive and physical function [29, 30], one of the biggest challenges is to identify strategies to develop and maintain functional ability at later ages. Functional ability is determined by the individual's intrinsic capacity, which encompasses cognitive function and mobility, relevant contextual factors, and the interaction between the two [7]. There is evidence that a physically active lifestyle and, consequently, a high level of functional fitness are effective modifiable risk factors that may slow the increase of cognitive impairments in older age [31–33].

Therefore, from a healthy aging perspective, an early intervention strategy based on supportive environments and opportunities to increase physical activities are determinants of living a long and healthy life [7]. This is supported by physical activity being a modifiable risk factor for cognitive impairment in older age [32, 33]. For this reason, in the last decade, there has been a rapid increase in interest in the potential of physical activity to prevent cognitive decline and maintain good cognitive abilities.

Although it has been demonstrated that maintenance of higher levels of physical activity helps to protect against cognitive deterioration, even at an advanced age [34, 35], it is still an open question which frequency, intensity, time, type, volume, and progression of physical activity is more effective to improve cognition. Finally, the physiological mechanisms underlying the relationship between cognitive function, functional fitness, and physical activity at older ages are still poorly understood.

4.2 Physical activity, well-being, and health-related quality of life

Observational studies have shown an average 20 to 30% reduction in mortality risk when individuals spend at least 1000 kcal per week on physical activity [36]. The American College of Sports Medicine emphasizes the health benefits associated with higher levels of physical activity and aerobic exercise across physiological, metabolic, and psychological parameters. Additionally, there is a decreased risk of many chronic diseases and premature mortality. The variables studied show a lower risk for any cause of mortality in people who maintain higher levels of physical activity or physical fitness over time when compared to those who reduce or maintain low levels of physical activity or physical fitness over time [37, 38].

Some recognized benefits of participating in regular physical activity are slowing physiologic changes of aging that impair exercise capacity [37], optimizing age-related changes in body composition [13], promoting psychological and cognitive well-being [20, 39], managing chronic diseases [40], reducing the risks of physical disability [25], and increasing longevity [41].

Despite the benefits of PA, older adults are the least physically active of all age groups, with only 11% of individuals aged ≥65 yrs engaging in aerobic and muscle-strengthening activities that meet guidelines, and less than 5% of individuals aged 85 yrs and older meet the same guidelines [37, 38].

5. Topic 4: contextual determinants of physical activity in the elderly population adopting and maintaining physically active lifestyle

5.1 Adoption and maintenance of physically active lifestyles

Some physical activity is better than none, and an increase in the physical activity level, up to a point, is better than less. This supports the dose-response relationship between physical activity and health reported by the American College of Sports Medicine in conjunction with other important health organizations such as the Centers for Disease Control and Prevention (CDC), the US Surgeon General, and the National Institutes of Health [42]. The main purpose of healthcare professionals and physical activity instructors is to assist individuals in adopting and adhering to the exercise prescription recommendations made throughout the guidelines. And the main challenge is to overcome the barriers to the exercise.

There are well-known correlates that affect engagement in regular physical activity. Numerous demographic factors (e.g. age, gender, socioeconomic status, education, and ethnicity) are consistently related to the likelihood that an individual will keep their activity regularly [43, 44].

In the context of adopting and maintaining a physically active lifestyle in older people, it is important to focus on the role that modifiable factors have on exercise prescription recommendations, the behavioral theories and models that have been applied to enhance exercise adoption and maintenance, and behavioral strategies and approaches that can be used to increase physical activity behaviors.

Physical activity tends to decline with age, especially when people have age-related disabilities. Still, age does not necessarily predispose an individual to lower activity [45]. Several international studies provide insights on impediments to physical activity in older people. The most common barriers reported were enough other hobbies, too exhausting, risk of injury too high, no knowledge of opportunities, an attitude that sports are only for younger people, no time, and financial reasons, having too few friends to exercise with [46]. Pain is another common barrier to exercise [47]. Another critical point concerns the differences between men and women, reinforcing the importance of specific efforts to increase older adults' physical activity levels [46]. We recognized that it is crucial, in each context, to identify earlier relevant barriers to physical activity in older adults to better tailor measures to the specific needs and be successful in the promotion and intervention strategies.

People's physical activity during their leisure time is determined by genetic traits (20 to 70&), beliefs and motivation shaped by learning (25 to 75%), and physical and social environments (10 to 50%) [45]. Creating a friendly-environment that makes physical activity easy/affordable does not ensure that a person living in that environment will be motivated to use it. It is not easy to alter personal preferences or long-standing habits. Changing physical activity is not like changing most other behaviors.

Sustained participation in regular physical activity requires active behavior modification. Following [45] in the "physical activity epidemiology," most behavior modification techniques for changing physical activity center on (i) goal-setting based on personal characteristics; (ii) identification of personal costs and expected barriers to adoption and maintenance of an activity routine; (iii) strategies for preventing or minimizing the impact of barriers to participation and for increasing support and reinforcement from friends and family; (iv) planning a gradual progression of difficulty to optimize success so that the participant has growing confidence in both physical abilities and the ability to maintain the new pattern of activity; (v) feedback from fitness testing and self-monitoring of activity and progress by the participant; and (vi) personal strategies for returning to activity after relapse to inactivity due to flagging motivation, injury, vacation, and others.

5.2 Age-friendly environments

Promoting age-friendly physical and social environments where people live plays a vital role in whether people can remain healthy, independent, and autonomous long into their old age [7].

Healthcare professionals and physical activity instructors have the responsibility to think correctly about the promotion of age-friendly environments. Promote age-friendly environments means offering free physical and social barriers and support policies, services, products, or technologies that help promote health and build and maintain physical and mental capacities across the life course. Also, age-friendly environments should enable people, even when experiencing capacity loss, to continue to do the things they value. When planning age-friendly practices, healthcare professionals and physical activity instructors must ensure that they are promoting/offering opportunities for older people to meet their basic needs, learn, grow, and make decisions, be mobile, build and maintain relationships, and contribute to the community.

Good practices of Age-Friendly Communities are well documented. For example, the 2022–2027 Master Aging Plan marks the fifth strategic planning cycle for the Orange County Department on Aging [48]. This Master Aging Plan framework contains eight domains of livability that influence the quality of life for older adults: (1) outdoor spaces and buildings (include actions to optimize usability of outdoor spaces and buildings); (ii) transportation (include actions to increase access to and awareness of affordable, safe, and equitable mobility options); (iii) housing (include actions to improve choice, quality, affordability, and stability of housing); (iv) social participation (include actions to promote diverse and accessible opportunities for participation and engagement); (V) respect and social inclusion (include actions to uphold all older adults ages 55+ years as valuable members and provide equitable resources for the community); (vi) civic participation and employment (include actions to connect older adults with resources that help them achieve their diverse employment and career transition goals); (vii) communication and information (include actions to awareness of and access to available services and supports for older adults and their families will increase for everyone), and (viii) community and health services (include actions to ensure the community has accessible and affordable resources to support individual health and well-being goals throughout the aging process). This plan builds off of the 20-year history of formal age-friendly planning in Orange County. This is a model for comprehensive and successful aging and represents a comprehensive vision for the future of several communities that intend to be age-friendly communities.

6. Topic 5: exercise prescription in the elderly population

6.1 Pre-exercise assessment

When people are encouraged to engage in physical activity because of its multiple health benefits, attempts to reduce the risks inherent in more vigorous activities should be considered. Screening for risk factors and/or symptoms of cardiovascular, pulmonary, and metabolic diseases, as well as other conditions (e.g. musculoskeletal conditions), may be aggravated by exercise [38]. The primary goals of pre-participation health screening and risk stratification are to help develop an effective and safe exercise prescription and optimize safety during exercise assessment and performance.

A health screening before starting an exercise or physical activity program is a tiered process: (i) self-guided method via the Physical Activity Readiness Questionnaire (PAR-Q) or the modified AHA/ACSM Health/Fitness Facility Questionnaire Preparticipation; (ii) assessment of risk factors for CVD and classification; and (iii) medical evaluation, including physical examinations and stress tests.

All older people who wish to start a physical activity program should be assessed at least through a medical history or self-reported health risk questionnaire; the responses to these self-guided methods determine the need and level of follow-up.

Older adults at moderate risk with two or more cardiovascular risk factors should be encouraged to consult a physician before starting a program of vigorous-intensity physical activity. Although medical evaluation is ongoing, most individuals can begin light to moderate-intensity exercise programs without consulting their physician. Older people at high risk with symptoms or diagnosed illnesses should consult their physician before starting a physical activity and/or exercise program.

Routine stress tests are recommended for individuals at high risk, including those with a diagnosis of cardiovascular disease, symptoms suggestive of new or unstable cardiovascular disease, diabetes mellitus, cardiovascular risk factors, advanced kidney disease, and specific lung diseases.

These recommendations reduce the barriers to adopting more active lifestyles because most of the risks associated with exercise can be lessened by adopting a progressive exercise training regimen. Generally, there is a low risk of participating in physical activity programs.

The assessment of the functional fitness of older adults is of particular importance. First of all, it can be used to identify at-risk participants. Many independent older adults, often due to their sedentary lifestyles, function dangerously close to their maximum ability level during normal activities. Climbing stairs or getting out of a chair requires near maximum effort for many older individuals [30]. More than one-third of community-dwelling older adults are at risk for mobility problems and falls [49]. Early identification of physical decline and appropriate interventions could help to prevent functional impairments, such as in walking and stair climbing, that often result in falls and physical frailty [30].

Second, assessing functional fitness for better program planning and evaluation is essential. A comprehensive functional fitness test provides specific information regarding a client's physical strength and weaknesses associated with functional tasks and activity goals important to everyday living. This information is necessary to design individualized, targeted exercise, or physical activity programs for clients. Baseline measures repeated during the program provide critical data to track clients' progress, make program adjustments, provide personalized feedback, and evaluate program effectiveness.

6.2 Exercise programs for the older population

There are important considerations for exercise programming in older people that must be considered at the beginning to maximize the effective development of an exercise program [38].

First, the intensity and duration of physical activity should be light at the beginning, particularly for older adults who are highly deconditioned, functionally limited or have chronic conditions that affect their ability to perform physical tasks. The intensity must be controlled not only by the use of a subjective effort scale but also by a pain scale. Respecting the pain limit is fundamental to ensure continuity in the practice of physical exercise. Second, the progression of physical activity should be individualized and tailored to tolerance and preference. A conservative approach may be necessary for older adults who are highly deconditioned or physically limited to prevent injury events.

A significant and well-documented age-related associated decline is muscular strength, especially after 50 yrs. [50]. This decline is directly connected with loss of strength due to the atrophy of muscle fibers, with a preferential incidence in type II fibers [51]. Practically, this supports the importance of including resistance training across the lifespan since it becomes more critical with increasing age. Strength training involves using selected machines or free weights. Initial training sessions should be supervised and monitored by personnel sensitive to the special needs of older adults.

Once power training is the muscle fitness component that rapidly declines with aging and has been associated with a greater risk of accidental falls, older people benefit from this training. Some recommendations are underlined by ACSM, including single- and multiple-joint exercises (one to three sets) using light-to-moderate loading (30–60% of 1-RM) for 6–10 repetitions with high velocity.

Individuals with sarcopenia, defined as a progressive and widespread skeletal muscle disorder involving loss of muscle mass and function, are associated with several adverse outcomes including falls, functional decline, frailty, and mortality [52]. Sarcopenia has been considered a public health problem, affecting most older people and making them more vulnerable to falls [53]. For this reason, it is essential to increase muscular strength before older people are physiologically capable of engaging in aerobic training.

Another important recommendation for all older people, even if chronic conditions preclude activity at the recommended minimum amount, is that older adults should perform physical activity as tolerated to avoid being sedentary. Older people should gradually exceed the recommended minimum amounts of physical activity and attempt continued progression if they desire to improve and/or maintain their functional fitness. It is an important message for older people to inform them to exceed the recommended minimum amounts of physical activity to improve the management of chronic diseases and health conditions for which a higher level of physical activity is already known to confer a therapeutic benefit, for example, diabetes, blood pressure, obesity, depression, and other.

Regarding older people with identified cognitive declines, moderate-intensity physical activity should be encouraged. In the case of significant cognitive impairment, individualized assistance may require during the physical activity program.

Generically, ACSM recommends a structured physical activity session, with an appropriate cool-down, particularly among individuals with cardiovascular disease. The cool-down should include a gradual reduction of effort and intensity and, optimally, flexibility exercises.

It is high recommendable that the incorporation of behavioral strategies such as social support, self-efficacy, the ability to make healthy choices, and perceived safety all may enhance participation in a regular exercise program. In addition, older people should be provided with regular feedback, positive reinforcement, and other behavioral/programmatic strategies to enhance adherence. These final recommendations will better contribute to a more consistent healthy aging program.

Author details

Élvio Rúbio Gouveia[1,2,3*], Bruna R. Gouveia[3,4,5], Adilson Marques[6,7,8], Priscila Marconcin[8,9] and Andreas Ihle[3,10,11]

1 Department of Physical Education and Sport, University of Madeira, Funchal, Portugal

2 Laboratory of Robotics and Systems in Engineering and Science (LARSyS), Interactive Technologies Institute, Funchal, Portugal

3 Center for the Interdisciplinary Study of Gerontology and Vulnerability, University of Geneva, Geneva, Switzerland

4 Regional Directorate of Health, Secretary of Health of the Autonomous Region of Madeira, Funchal, Portugal

5 Saint Joseph of Cluny Higher School of Nursing, Funchal, Portugal

6 Interdisciplinary Centre for the Study of Human Performance (CIPER), Faculty of Human Kinetics, University of Lisbon, Lisbon, Portugal

7 Instituto de Saúde Ambiental (ISAMB), University of Lisbon, Lisbon, Portugal

8 Faculty of Human Kinetics, University of Lisbon, Lisbon, Portugal

9 KinesioLab, Research Unit in Human Movement Analysis, Piaget Institute, Almada, Portugal

10 Department of Psychology, University of Geneva, Geneva, Switzerland

11 Swiss National Centre of Competence in Research LIVES—Overcoming Vulnerability: Life Course Perspectives, Lausanne, Switzerland

*Address all correspondence to: erubiog@staff.uma.pt

References

[1] World Health Organization. Ageing and Health. Geneva: WHO Press; 2021. Accessed at: https://www.who.int/news-room/fact-sheets/detail/ageing-and-health

[2] Spirduso WW, Francis KL, MacRae PG. Physical Dimensions of Aging. Second ed. Champaign, IL: Human Kinetics; 2005

[3] Taylor AW, Johnson MJ. Physiology of Exercise and Healthy Aging. Champaign, IL: Human Kinetics; 2008

[4] Davidovic M, Sevo G, Svorcan P, Milosevic DP, Despotovic N, Erceg P. Old age as a privilege of the "selfish ones". Aging and Disease. 2010;**1**(2):139-146

[5] Jones CJ. Predictors of successful aging. In: Jones CJ, Rose DJ, editors. Physical Activity Instruction of Older Adults. Champaign, IL: Human Kinetics; 2005. pp. 11-21

[6] Jin K. Modern biological theories of aging. Aging and Disease. 2010;**1**(2):72-74

[7] World Health Organization. World Report on Ageing and Health. Geneva: WHO Press; 2015

[8] Schaap LA, van Schoor NM, Lips P, Visser M. Associations of sarcopenia definitions, and their components, with the incidence of recurrent falling and fractures: The longitudinal aging study Amsterdam. The Journals of Gerontology. Series A, Biological Sciences and Medical Sciences. 2018;**73**(9):1199-1204. DOI: 10.1093/gerona/glx245

[9] Bahat G, Ilhan B. Sarcopenia and the cardiometabolic syndrome: A narrative review. European Geriatric Medicine. 2016;**7**(3):220-223

[10] Bone AE, Hepgul N, Kon S, Maddocks M. Sarcopenia and frailty in chronic respiratory disease. Chronic Respiratory Disease. 2017;**14**(1):85-99. DOI: 10.1177/1479972316679664

[11] De Buyser SL, Petrovic M, Taes YE, Toye KR, Kaufman JM, Lapauw B, et al. Validation of the FNIH sarcopenia criteria and SOF frailty index as predictors of long-term mortality in ambulatory older men. Age and Ageing. 2016;**45**(5):602-608. DOI: 10.1093/ageing/afw071

[12] Visser M, Schaap LA. Consequences of sarcopenia. Clinics in Geriatric Medicine. 2011;**27**(3):387-399. DOI: 10.1016/j.cger.2011.03.006

[13] Gouveia ÉR, Gouveia BR, Maia JA, Blimkie CJ, Freitas DL. Skeletal muscle and physical activity in Portuguese community-dwelling older adults. Journal of Aging and Physical Activity. 2016;**24**(4):567-574. DOI: 10.1123/japa.2015-0129

[14] Aagaard P, Suetta C, Caserotti P, Magnusson SP, & Kjaer M. Role of the nervous system in sarcopenia and muscle atrophy with aging: Strength training as a countermeasure. Scandinavian Journal of Medicine & Science in Sports. 2010;**20**(1):49-64. DOI: 10.1111/j.1600-0838.2009.01084.x

[15] Baumgartner RN. Body composition in healthy aging. Annals of the New York Academy of Sciences. 2000;**904**:437-448. DOI: 10.1111/j.1749-6632.2000.tb06498.x

[16] Chodzko-Zajko WJ, Moore KA. Physical fitness and cognitive

functioning in aging. Exercise and Sport Sciences Reviews. 1994;**22**:195-220

[17] Gouveia ÉR, Smailagic A, Ihle A, Marques A, Gouveia BR, Cameirão M, et al. The efficacy of a multicomponent functional fitness program based on exergaming on cognitive functioning of healthy older adults: A randomized controlled trial. Journal of Aging and Physical Activity. 2021;**29**(4):586-594. DOI: 10.1123/japa.2020-0083

[18] Bherer L, Erickson KI, Liu-Ambrose T. A review of the effects of physical activity and exercise on cognitive and brain functions in older adults. Journal of Aging Research. 2013;**2013**:657508. DOI: 10.1155/2013/657508

[19] Northey JM, Cherbuin N, Pumpa, KL, Smee DJ, Rattray B. Exercise interventions for cognitive function in adults older than 50: A systematic review with meta-analysis. British Journal of Sports Medicine. 2018;**52**(3):154-160. DOI: 10.1136/bjsports-2016-096587

[20] Ihle A, Gouveia ÉR, Gouveia BR, van der Linden B, Sauter J, Gabriel R, et al. The role of leisure activities in mediating the relationship between physical health and well-being: Differential patterns in old and very old age. Gerontology. 2017;**63**(6):560-571. DOI: 10.1159/000477628

[21] Ballesteros S, Kraft E, Santana, S, Tziraki C. Maintaining older brain functionality: A targeted review. Neuroscience and Biobehavioral Reviews. 2015;**55**:453-477. DOI: 10.1016/j.neubiorev.2015.06.008

[22] Fernández-Ballesteros R. Envejecimiento Activo: Contribuciones de la Psicología. Madrid: Ediciones Pirámide; 2009

[23] Rikli RE, Jones CJ. senior fitness test manual. Development and Validation of a Functional Fitness Test for Community-Residing Older Adults. Champaign, IL: Human Kinetics; 2001

[24] Rikli RE, Jones CJ. Functional fitness normative scores for community-residing older adults, ages 60-94. Journal of Aging and Physical Activity. 1999;**7**:162

[25] Gouveia ÉR, Maia JA, Beunen GP, Blimkie CJ, Fena EM, Freitas DL. Functional fitness and physical activity of Portuguese community-residing older adults. Journal of Aging and Physical Activity. 2013;**21**(1):1-19. DOI: 10.1123/japa.21.1.1

[26] Krause MP, Januário RS, Hallage T, Haile L, Miculis CP, Gama MP, et al. A comparison of functional fitness of older Brazilian and American women. Journal of Aging and Physical Activity. 2009;**17**:387-397

[27] Ignasiak Zofia, Sebastjan Anna, SÅawiÅ„ska Teresa, Skrzek Anna, Czarny Wojciech, KrÃ3l PaweÅ„ Rzepko Marian, Duda-Biernacka Barbara, Marchewka Anna, Filar-Mierzwa Katarzyna, Nowacka-Dobosz Sylwia, Dobosz Janusz, Umiastowska Danuta (2020). Functional fitness normative values for elderly polish population. BMC Geriatrics, 20(1), 384. doi:10.1186/s12877-020-01787-2

[28] Zhao Y, Wang Z, Chung P-K, Wang S. Functional fitness norms and trends of community-dwelling older adults in urban China. Scientific Reports. 2021;**11**(1):17745. DOI: 10.1038/s41598-021-97320-5

[29] Glisky EL. Changes in cognitive function in human aging. In: Riddle DR, editor. Brain Aging: Models, Methods, and Mechanisms. Boca Raton (FL): CRC Press/Taylor & Francis; 2007

[30] Rikli RE, Jones CJ. Senior Fitness Test Manual. Champaign, IL: Human Kinetics, Inc; 2013

[31] Blondell SJ, Hammersley-Mather R, Veerman JL. Does physical activity prevent cognitive decline and dementia?: A systematic review and meta-analysis of longitudinal studies. BMC Public Health. 2014;**14**:510. DOI: 10.1186/1471-2458-14-510

[32] Barnes DE, Yaffe K. The projected effect of risk factor reduction on Alzheimer's disease prevalence. The Lancet Neurology. 2011;**10**(9):819-828. DOI: 10.1016/s1474-4422(11)70072-2

[33] Deckers K, van Boxtel MPJ, Schiepers OJG, de Vugt M, Sánchez M, Luis J, et al. Target risk factors for dementia prevention: A systematic review and Delphi consensus study on the evidence from observational studies. International Journal of Geriatric Psychiatry. 2015;**30**(3):234-246. DOI: 10.1002/gps.4245

[34] Stubbs B, Vancampfort D, Rosenbaum S, Firth J, Cosco T, Veronese N, et al. An examination of the anxiolytic effects of exercise for people with anxiety and stress-related disorders: A meta-analysis. Psychiatry Research. 2017;**249**:102-108. DOI: 10.1016/j.psychres.2016.12.020

[35] Umegaki H, Makino T, Uemura K, Shimada H, Cheng XW, Kuzuya M. Objectively measured physical activity and cognitive function in urban-dwelling older adults. Geriatrics & Gerontology International. 2018;**18**(6):922-928. DOI: 10.1111/ggi.13284

[36] Dishman RK, Washburn RA, Heath GW. Physical Activity Epidemiology. Champaign, IL: Human Kinetics; 2004

[37] Izquierdo M, Merchant RA, Morley JE, Anker SD, Aprahamian I, Arai H, et al. International exercise recommendations in older adults (ICFSR): Expert consensus guidelines. The Journal of Nutrition, Health & Aging. 2021;**25**(7):824-853. DOI: 10.1007/s12603-021-1665-8

[38] Liguori G. American College of Sports Medicine. ACSM's Guidelines for Exercise Testing and Prescription. Philadelphia: Lippincott Williams & Wilkins; 2020

[39] Gouveia É, Gouveia BR, Ihle A, Kliegel M, Maia JA, Badia I, et al. Correlates of health-related quality of life in young-old and old-old community-dwelling older adults. Quality of Life Research: an International Journal of Quality of Life Aspects of Treatment, Care and Rehabilitation. 2017b;**26**(6):1561-1569. DOI: 10.1007/s11136-017-1502-z

[40] Gouveia ÉR, Ihle A, Kliegel M, Freitas DL, Jurema J, Tinôco MA, et al. The relationship of physical activity to high-density lipoprotein cholesterol level in a sample of community-dwelling older adults from Amazonas, Brazil. Archives of Gerontology and Geriatrics. 2017c;**73**:195-198. DOI: 10.1016/j.archger.2017.08.004

[41] Partridge L, Deelen J, Slagboom PE. Facing up to the global challenges of ageing. Nature. 2018;**561**(7721):45-56. DOI: 10.1038/s41586-018-0457-8

[42] Geidl W, Schlesinger S, Mino E, Miranda L, Pfeifer K. Dose-response relationship between physical activity and mortality in adults with noncommunicable diseases: A systematic review and meta-analysis of prospective observational studies. The International Journal of Behavioral Nutrition and

Physical Activity. 2020;**17**(1):109. DOI: 10.1186/s12966-020-01007-5

[43] Bauman AE, Reis RS, Sallis JF, Wells JC, Loos RJ, Martin BW, et al. Correlates of physical activity: Why are some people physically active and others not? Lancet (London, England). 2012;**380**(9838):258-271

[44] Macera CA, Ham SA, Yore MM, Jones DA, Ainsworth BE, Kimsey CD, et al. Prevalence of physical activity in the United States: Behavioral risk factor surveillance system, 2001. Preventing Chronic Disease. 2005;**2**(2):A17

[45] Dishman RK, Heath GW, Lee I-M. Physical Activity Epidemiology. 2nd edition. Champaign, IL: Human Kinetics; 2013

[46] Moschny A, Platen P, Klaassen-Mielke R, Trampisch U, Hinrichs T. Barriers to physical activity in older adults in Germany: A cross-sectional study. The International Journal of Behavioral Nutrition and Physical Activity. 2011;**8**:121. DOI: 10.1186/1479-5868-8-121

[47] Vader K, Doulas T, Patel R, Miller J. Experiences, barriers, and facilitators to participating in physical activity and exercise in adults living with chronic pain: A qualitative study. Disability and Rehabilitation. 2021;**43**(13):1829-1837

[48] Tyler J, Wood K, Dictus C. Orange county - master aging plan 2022-2027. 2022. Accessed in https://extranet.who.int/agefriendlyworld/wp-content/uploads/2022/06/Final-2022-27-MASTER-AGING-PLAN-8.5x11.pdf

[49] Rose DJ. Fall Proof: A Comprehensive Balance and Mobility Training Program, 2nd ed. Champaign IL: Human Kinetics; 2010

[50] Keller K, Engelhardt M. Strength and muscle mass loss with aging process. Age and strength loss. Muscles, Ligaments and Tendons Journal. 2013;**3**:346-350. PubMed ID: 24596700. DOI: 10.32098/mltj.04.2013.17

[51] Rice J, Keogh JW. Power training: Can it improve functional performance in older adults? A systematic review. International Journal of Exercise Science. 2009;**2**:131-151

[52] Cruz-Jentoft AJ, Bahat G, Bauer J, Boirie Y, Bruyère O, Cederholm T, et al. Sarcopenia: Revised European consensus on definition and diagnosis. Age and Ageing. 2019;**48**(1):16-31. DOI: 10.1093/ageing/afy169

[53] Pelegrini A, Mazo GZ, Pinto AdA, Benedetti TRB, Silva DAS, Petroski EL. Sarcopenia: Prevalence and associated factors among elderly from a Brazilian capital. Fisioterapia em Movimento. 2018;**31**:e003102. DOI:10.1590/1980-5918.031.ao02

Chapter 3

Perspective Chapter: Geriatric Care in Africa

Dabota Yvonne Buowari

Abstract

There are an increasing number of people that are aging. This is also common in Africa. Therefore, they need specialist care from various categories of health care workers and other professionals on geriatric medicine and gerontology. There are few geriatricians in Africans. This is because there are few training centres in the continents. Also, most of the geriatricians are trained on the other side of the continent overseas.

Keywords: Africa, geriatric medicine, gerontology, population, aging

1. Introduction

As human beings are born, the aging process begins. There are many phases of life from being a neonate, infant toddler, adolescent, teenager, young adult, youth and then old age. As people age, there are challenges and problems associated with aging including health. The health needs of the elderly need to be cared for by medical doctors specially trained to care for the elderly persons who require special communication skills. Old age is a period in the lives of the elderly for rest after a long life of activity and service [1]. In some communities and societies, socio-cultural referents are used to define old age such as family status if the person has become a grandparent, physical appearances such as the appearance of gray hair and wrinkles [2].

Geriatric medicine is still a new medical specialty in most parts of the world; like any other career choice, there are still gaps in the knowledge, awareness and uptake as a profession [3, 4]. The elderly face a lot of challenges [5] physically, medically, socially, economically and otherwise. Geriatric medicine differs from typical adult medicine because it focuses specifically on the unique needs and health challenges of older adult [6]. There is generally a paucity of specialized healthcare services for the elderly in Africa, some of the reasons may be lack of training in most African countries, unawareness of the peculiar needs of the elderly and lack of human and material resources [7]. Geriatric medicine is important because most doctors deal with elderly patients no matter their specialty [8, 9].

Globally, the population is aging. It is therefore necessary that aged persons are healthy and physically active [10]. This longevity is due to several factors such as good sanitation, access to good healthcare, more people are getting educated, healthy eating and access to funds to provide the necessities of life. Some persons may become less physically active when they age. However, there is a connection between being less physically active and becoming frail [11]. Aging takes place throughout the lifetime, as it creates an opportunity to improve and preserve the physical, health, mental well-being and improve the quality of life. The aging of the population leads to various challenges, which may be economic and social. Also, the health of the person getting older may be affected as the elderly is predisposed to certain illnesses. Governments globally need to set up the right policies that will address the challenges faced by the aged [11]. Some senior citizens are discriminated against in their communities in Africa especially if they are women and childless. Other social challenges senior citizens encounter in Africa are social isolation, elder abuse, neglect and abandonment. This is common because nursing homes and long-term care facilities are not common in Africa. Even in communities where they are available, they are underutilized. Geriatric care cannot be complete without the provision of long-term care facilities [12]. The populace needs to be educated and enlightened on the need for long-term care [12]. This is because the long-term care will provide relief for family members who have elderly persons that are frail or cannot carry out the activities of daily living by themselves or need assistance. Elderly persons in Africa generally encounter several difficulties in which their health, well-being and mental state are affected [13]. This is due to health system inadequacies and lack of care for older persons and unavailable long-term care facilities for older persons. Older persons in Africa are well respected [14]. Older women perform other roles in Africa especially carrying for their grandchildren especially if the mother of their grandchildren has passed away [14]. They are employed as babysitters and nannies. Sometimes they travel overseas to care for their grandchildren so that their children can go to work and not pay for child care.

As times are changing, many young people are getting formal employment, there will be an increased demand for long-term care facilities inform of nursing homes to care for the elderly [12]. This will help the elderly to maintain good health and access social support. Though, even the available nursing homes in some African communities are underutilized. This is due to several factors, people are not aware of their existence, beliefs and myths about nursing homes and discrimination and humiliation of people who take their elderly ones to nursing homes [15]. Some of the nursing homes in Africa are managed by religious organizations. In Africa, elders are cared for by their offspring, grandchildren and extended family members [12, 14].

2. Population aging

Population aging is a worldwide phenomenon with economic and social consequences, and it follows a decline in both birth and death rates [5, 16–20]. Globally, there is an increase in the number of elderly persons who will require geriatric care [5, 8, 17, 18, 21–30]. They make up a large number of the population in every country. This worldwide increase in the number of aged persons will increase the importance of the geriatric medicine specialty [26]. This is because old age comes with certain challenges, and chronic illnesses will become a major global public health challenge [19]. The increase in longevity is linked to the reduction in the death rate due to improved health systems and interventions [18, 28, 31].

Globally in 2017, the number of persons aged 60 years and above was 962 million, and this figure is expected to double by 2015 [2, 18, 20]. Population aging will have an impact on healthcare delivery both positively and negatively as there will be a shift from acute to chronic diseases associated with old age and the likelihood of a shortage of healthcare workers specially trained to look after the aged [19, 32, 33]. Like any other group of individuals in society, the aged require constant interaction with people around them [5]. Generally, in most societies and cultures including Africa, it is expected that older people are relieved from normal labour and allowed rest from active economic activities [1]. The aging population is of great concern for the health sector as health challenges are common among the elderly [17, 34] with different patterns of presentation which therefore requires special medical skills [8, 35].

3. Demography of elderly persons in Africa

It is not news that there are older persons in Africa. Worldwide, it is estimated in 2019 that there were 1 billion persons who are 60 years and above [36]. However it is estimated that this number will rise to 2 billion by 2050, there is also speculation that there shall also be an increase in the number of people that will live up to 80 years and beyond [37]. The number of older persons is increasing dramatically, especially in countries that are still developing. Most of which are African countries [38]. It is estimated by the United Nations that by the year 2045, there will be more people that will be over the age of 65 years which will outnumber the number of persons that will be below 15 years [38]. Older persons in recent times consist of a significantly larger population. In Africa, it was estimated in 2009 that 53.8 million individuals are aged 60 years and above [38]. Generally, few persons are trained in geriatric medicine and gerontology to care for the aging population in Africa.

4. Who is an elder?

The elderly are also known as senior citizens, the aged, older persons and elder statesmen. There is no precise and accurate definition of who is an elder [39] as there are different definitions for the elderly by several international organizations, and it varies from society to society [40]. The United Nations agreed that the cut-off age for an older person is someone who is 60 years and above [1, 2, 41], while the World Health Organization defines an elder to be 65 years and above [42, 43]. Most developed countries have accepted the chronological age of 65 years as a definition of elderly individuals [5, 42, 44]. In some countries, the definition of old age is linked to the age of retirement from the government civil service [5, 21]. For instance, the cut-off age for elderly persons in Nigeria is 60 years as this is the age for retirement from the Nigerian federal and state civil service. Though with the various definitions of old age or who is an elder, there is no general agreement on the age when a person becomes old [5].

5. Aging in Africa

Older persons play important roles in African societies as the African cultural systems give them high status [45]. They preserve cultural values, transmit knowledge and skills, dissolve conflicts and disagreements and also educate the young [2, 46]. The typical older adult in developing countries lives in poverty [7]. In some African countries, the kin of elderly people accuse them of witchcraft that they are the cause of misfortunes in the family [29]. This is worst for elderly women who do not have any living child; sometimes these older women are ostracized, tortured or even killed [29].

Over half of persons aged 60 years and above in Africa resided with a child either their biological children or grandchild [23] as the family and friends care for older persons [46]. Older persons in most African societies are accorded much respect [46]. Sometimes older persons are not called directly by their names. They are called mama, for women and papa or baba for men depending on the country. They are addressed as mothers or fathers irrespective of whether they have children or not. In Nigeria, there are different tribes and each tribe has a prefix added to the name of an older person. Among the Ibani people of Grand Bonny Kingdom and Opobo in Rivers State, Nigeria, the prefix 'Ada' is used for older men and 'Aya' for older women. Among the Igbo tribe of Eastern Nigeria, the prefix 'Dede' is used for older men and 'Dada' for older women. Baba is the prefix used for older men among the Yoruba people of Western Nigeria. It is an insult and also seen as a sign of disrespect in most African countries to address an older person directly by their names. The respect of older persons is also seen in several cultures including greeting and acknowledging them. For instance, among the Ibani tribe of southern Nigeria, a man must remove his hat when greeting an elder especially if the older is a man. Among the Yoruba, an older person is greeted by a female kneeling down or a male prostrating on the ground. This shows that Africans hold the older person in high esteem and these traditions have been passed down from generation to generation.

In Africa, the chronological definition of the older person sometimes causes some problems as due to illiteracy, most dates of birth are not recorded [5, 40]. Sometimes historic events are used to estimate the age. In some African countries, aging is associated with retirement and the receipt of pension [1]. Though not all African older persons have been involved in formal work, older persons in Africa are involved in transmitting oral, culture and traditions from one generation to another [2]. In Africa and other countries, senior citizens may be perceived as burdens due to their disability or dependence [21].

The elderly also known as older persons or senior citizens are persons aged 60 years and over [47]. Some others define the elderly as persons aged 65 years and above. In Nigeria, 60 years is used as this is the age of retirement from the Nigerian government civil service. Few other professionals in Africa retire above the age of 60 such as judges and lecturers.

Elderly persons are well respected as they are believed to be full of wisdom. During family and community conflicts, they are made head of locally constituted panels to deliberate on issues that range from marriage disputes, sibling rivalry and land disputes. Their verdicts are respected and taken as the final even if the decision is not reasonable. Most elderly persons in Africa do not have any form of pension or retirement benefits. They are cared for by their family members who are their biological children, nephews and nieces, community members and sometimes members of religious organizations. Therefore, they need social support as this will in turn affect their health and psychological well-being, mental health, quality of life, independence, interpersonal relationship and personality [48]. This is because social support will reduce boredom and loneliness. There will also be a reduction in elder abuse, neglect and mental health problems such as anxiety and depression.

In sub-Saharan Africa, most elderly women are not unemployed, therefore, they do not benefit from any form of social security, and hence, they are vulnerable [13]. Older persons in Africa are sometimes accused as the cause of misfortunes that happens or is experienced by their siblings and sibling children, especially if the older person is a woman and childless.

Older persons tend to retire to their rural areas and villages when they retire from formal employment. Social amenities of life are absent in most African villages such as electricity, good pipe bore water and in recent times the internet and mobile telecommunication services. They do not have access to healthcare when they retire to the village as most of the healthcare facilities in Africa are located in urban areas and cities. The elderly are sometimes termed as witches and wizards that possess spiritual powers to inflict evil on whomsoever they want.

6. Education and training in geriatric medicine in Africa

Doctors who are specialists in geriatric medicine are known as geriatricians. There are few hospitals in Africa that provide special care for the elderly with a unit division or department of geriatric medicine. Such units are manned by doctors who have either trained abroad either in Europe or the United States of America in geriatric medicine or generalist either internal medicine physicians or family doctors with interest in caring for the elderly. There is a dilemma in Africa if generalists with an interest in caring for the elderly should be referred to as geriatricians.

Globally, there are few geriatricians. In a study among medical graduates to find out those interested in geriatrics in medical schools in the United Kingdom, only 0.9% (0.4% males, 1.3% females) after 1 year of qualification and 1.5% (1.2% males, 1.9%) females after 5 years were interested in becoming geriatricians [26].

Geriatrics is not relatively popular among medical students [9], especially in Africa where most medical students are not even exposed to geriatric medicine in medical school. In another study in South Africa, only 6.6% wanted to specialize in geriatric medicine [16].

Geriatric medicine is a relatively new medical subspecialty in most parts of the world including Africa [16, 49]. It is complex to train as a geriatrician [50]. Unlike many other physicians who have a high proportion of older patients in their practice, geriatricians place a high premium on improving the function of their patients and not just treating the disease [51]. Globally, there are several models of specialty training to become a geriatrician [6]. Some doctors enrol in residency training in geriatric medicine. Another career pathway is to complete the residency in either internal medicine or family medicine depending on what is obtainable in the country and then train in a 1 year clinical fellowship [6]. Another career pathway is to complete a postgraduate degree that is Diploma, Masters or Doctor of Philosophy (PhD) in geriatric medicine [6]. Another pathway which is that some African doctors have done is to write the diploma in geriatric medicine examination of the Royal College of Physicians of London. In Canada, only candidates certified by the Royal College of Physicians and Surgeons of Canada in internal medicine may be eligible for certification in geriatric medicine [52].

In most countries, geriatric medicine is hardly included in undergraduate training [16]. This may be due to the lack of geriatricians. Specialization in geriatric medicine has traditionally been within internal medicine but a trend in some countries is for geriatricians to be trained within family medicine [16]. Medical training should embrace a multidisciplinary perspective team with particular attention given to the special care needs of the elderly persons reflecting the fact that they include medical conditions unique to this age group [30]. Development of geriatric care should be enhanced in undergraduate and also at postgraduate levels of training [26]. A Diploma in Geriatric Medicine is awarded by the Royal College of Physicians of

London. The examination is designed to give recognition of competence in the provision of care of older people to general practitioners, trainees, middle-grade doctors working in non-consultant career posts in departments of geriatric medicine and other doctors with interest in or responsible for the care of older people [53]. Some Africans have passed this examination.

7. Geriatric care in Africa

Formalized care for the elderly is not adequate and well developed in Africa. There are few geriatricians in Africa including few training centres dedicated to the training for geriatric medicine. However, there are few training centres in African countries such as South Africa. In Nigeria, the training in geriatric medicine is still new and only a few hospitals are accredited by the West African College of Surgeons for the training of geriatricians in Africa. This is done after success in the junior residency emanations. Most geriatricians working in Africa have been trained overseas. In developed countries, some other doctors who have an interest in the care of the elderly but do not have the opportunity to have specialist training in geriatric medicine have attended refresher courses in geriatric medicine. There are family doctors and physicians who have gained their experience in geriatric medicine by interest in the specialty and devoting their time and energy to caring for the elderly. Most African societies are becoming urbanized, and this is affecting the care of older persons making them vulnerable, dissolution of the structure of the family and lack of access to good healthcare [13]. Even with experience in caring for older persons, their knowledge will be limited because they do not have any specialists training in geriatric medicine [38].

In a study conducted by Dotchin et al., on the services and training in geriatric medicine in Africa, in most African communities, there are limited specialist healthcare services for older persons [38]. Several medical specialties are encompassed in geriatric medicine such as family medicine, internal medicine, emergency medicine, surgery and dermatology. Geriatric medicine as a specialty is not taught in medical schools [38]. Governments in developing countries have an important role in the provision of healthcare for elder persons [12]. The governments need to enact policies and laws that will protect the vulnerability of senior citizens. Care of the elder citizens is not of importance to the policymakers in most African countries.

There are few geriatric centres or units in Africa. This may be because there are few training centres for geriatric medicine in Africa. In Nigeria, for instance, as at the time of writing this book, there is the Tony Anenih Geriatric Centre at the University College Hospital, Ibadan; Care of Elderly Person's Unit (CEPU) at the University of Port Harcourt Teaching Hospital and the Geriatric Unit at the University of Benin Teaching Hospital, Benin City, Edo State. The Geriatric Unit of the University of Benin Teaching Hospital was created in October; 2013 [7]. Other Nigerian hospitals have a special clinic for older persons but are not organized by the hospital management as a geriatric unit or department. In the face of limited resources, it is possible to establish a functional geriatric unit and achieve best practices in resource-limited settings by investing in improving available human resources and infrastructure [7].

In Nigeria, there is no organized training for geriatric medicine but doctors with an interest in caring for the elderly practice geriatric medicine and care for the health needs of the elderly. This includes family doctors and physicians. Anesthetists with an interest in geriatric medicine practise geriatric anesthesia. Few Nigerian doctors have trained to be geriatricians in the United Kingdom and the United States of America or have passed the diploma in geriatric medicine examination of the Royal College of Physicians. In March 2016, the University College Hospital, Ibadan, Nigeria, organized a 2 week certificate course on geriatric medicine to train family doctors and physicians in geriatric medicine. This introductory training to geriatric medicine has been done for some years after the maiden one.

Nursing homes are long-term care facilities for vulnerable groups of people for example children, motherless babies, the disabled, mentally retarded and the elderly. These are not common in Nigeria as most Nigerian nursing homes are established and managed by religious organizations and/or non-governmental organizations. Institutional homes for the elderly have their problems, therefore the residents need medical care. In Africa, due to the culture of the people, the elderly resist being kept in a home either as daycare or for long-term care instead they are to be taken care of by their children or other relatives [54]. This is also applicable to Nigeria as the Nigerian elderly are still cared for by their families [55]. One of the reasons why in countries such as Nigeria, the elderly person will not be kept in a long-term home is the belief that the elderly will place a curse on whoever brings the idea and support any placement in the long-term care facility or children or other family members [55].

Sometimes, some of the residents of the nursing homes are abandoned and neglected by their relatives. In this modern day, where young people both men and women have to be involved in circular work or businesses that keep them away from home, specialized long-term institutions are necessary to care for the vulnerable groups of people in the society including the elderly.

8. Conclusions

There are a rising number of people getting older and living up to 60 years and above. This group of people in Africa is faced with several challenges, and they are prone to vulnerability. They are faced with health and social problems. This is worst for women who are single as they are sometimes ostracized and even called witches. There are few geriatricians in Africa; however, most countries are developing strategies for various forms of training in geriatric medicine such as postgraduate courses, fellowship, refresher courses and workshops. There is need for more research on the elderly in Africa. The different states in the African continent should enact policies and laws to protect senior citizens in Africa.

Author details

Dabota Yvonne Buowari
Department of Accident and Emergency, University of Port Harcourt Teaching Hospital, Port Harcourt, Nigeria

*Address all correspondence to: dabotabuowari@yahoo.com

References

[1] Baloyi ME. A pastoral investigation into some of the challenges associated with ageing and retirement in the south African context. Indie Shriflig Art. 49 (3) Art # 1866. 10 pages. DOI: 10.4102/ids.v.49.3.1866

[2] United Nations High Commissioner for Refugees, The United Nations Refugee Agency. Working with Older Persons in Forced Displacement. Geneva. 2013. Retrieved from: www.unhcr.org. [Accessed: October 2019]

[3] Byszewski A, Bezzina K, Latrous M. What kind of doctor do you want to be? Geriatric medicine podcast as a career planning resource. Biomedical Resource International. 2017:1-6. DOI: 10.115/2017/618348

[4] Brubaker JK. The birtf a new specialty: Geriatrics. Journal of Lancaster General Hospital. 2008;**3**(3):105-107

[5] Abiodum MG, Adekeye OA, Iruonagbe TC. Counselling services for remediating the biopsychosocial challenges of the aged in Nigeria. Journal of Functional Management. 2011;**3**(1):89-98

[6] Won CW, Kim S, Swagerty D. Why geriatric medicine is important for Korea: Lessons learned in the United States. Journal of Korean Medical Science. 2018;**33**(26):e17. DOI: 10.3346/jkms.2018.33.e175

[7] Akoria OA. Establishing in-hospital geriatrics services in Africa: Insights from the University of Benin Teaching Hospital geriatrics project. Annals of African Medicine. 2016;**15**(3):145-153

[8] Cooper N, Forrest K, Muller G. ABC of Geriatric Medicine. 1st ed. Wiley; 2013. pp. 2-100

[9] Marjolein HJ, Joep L, Elise LK, Marcel GMO, Cornelia RMGF, Antonie LML. 2 lessons learned from narrative feedback of students on a geriatric training program. Gerontology and Geriatrics Education. 2018;**39**(1):21-34

[10] Naah FL, Njong AM, Kimengsi JN. Determinants of active and healthy ageing in sub-Saharan Africa: Evidence from Cameroon. International Journal of Environmental Research Public Health. 2020;**17**:3038. DOI: 10.3390/ijerph17093038

[11] Tanyi PL, Andre P, Mbah P. Care of the elderly in Nigeria: Policy implications. Legent Social Sciences. 2018;**4**(1):1555201. DOI: 10.1080/23311886.2018.155521

[12] Towards Long-Term Care Systems in Sub-Saharan Africa: WHO Series on Long-Term Care. Geneva: World Health Organization; 2017 Licence: CCBY-NC-SA30

[13] Parmar D, Williams G, Dkhimi F, Ndiaye A, Asante FA, Arhinful DK, et al. Enrolment of older people in social health protection programs in West Africa - does social exclusion play a part? Social Science and Medicine. 2014;**119**:36-44

[14] Dotchin CL, Akinyemi RO, Gray WK, Walker RW. Geriatric medicine, services and training in Africa. Age and Ageing Advance. 2012;**6**:1-9. DOI: 10.1093/ageing/afs119

[15] Help Age International. Discrimination against older women in Burkina Faso. Parallel Report Submitted to the 47th Session of the Committee on the Elimination of All Forms of Discrimination Against Women

(CEDAW) in relation to Burkina Faso's Sixth periodic report of States parties, CEDAW/C/BFA/6. 2009

[16] Ferreira M. Geriatric medicine in South Africa-a Cinderella subspecialty? South Africa Family Practice. 2008;**48**(8):18

[17] Sidik SM, Rampal L, Afifi M. Physical and mental health problems of the elderly in a rural community of Sepang. Selangor. Malaysian Journal of Medical Science. 2004;**11**(1):52-59

[18] Gerber AM, Mostert A, Botes R, Vorster A, Bustens E. A cohort study of elderly people in Bloemfontein, South Africa to determine health-related quality of life and functional abilities. South African Medical Journal. 2016;**106**(3):298-301

[19] Naja S, Makhlouf MMD, Chehab MAH. An ageing world of the 21st century: A literature review. International Journal of Community Medicine and Public Health. 2017;**4**(12):4363-4369

[20] D'Albis H, Collard F. Age groups and the measure of population ageing. Demographic Research. 2013;**29**(23):617-640 www.demographic-research.org assessed 2018

[21] Men Ageing and Health. Geneva: World Health Organization. www.who.int Assessed October 2018

[22] Karthaus M, Falkenstein M. Functional changes and driving performance in older drivers: Assessment and interventions. Geriatrics. 2016:1-18. DOI: 10.3396/geriatrics/020012. Available from: www.mdpi.com/journal/geriatrics [Accessed: October 2018]

[23] Department of Economic and Social Affairs, Population Division. World Population Ageing 2017 - Highlights (ST/ESA/SER.A/397). United Nations; 2017

[24] Asthana S, Golden RN. The ageing imperative - innovations in research, education and care in geriatric medicine. World Medical Journal. 2018;**117**:92-93

[25] Hajjar ER, Cafiero AC, Hanlon JT. Polypharmacy in elderly patients. The American Journal of Geriatric Pharmacotherapy. 2007;**5**:345-351

[26] Maisonneuve JJ, Pulford C, Lambert TW, Goldacre MJ. Career choices for geriatric medicine: National surveys for graduates of 1974 – 2009 from all UK medical schools. Age and Ageing. 2014;**43**:535-541

[27] Pillay NK, Maharaj P. Population ageing in Africa. In: Maharaj P, editor. Ageing and Health in Africa. International Perspectives on Aging. New York: Springer Science; 2013. pp. 11-51

[28] Chaudhary P, Lamba N. Critical review of geriatric care in Ayurveda with special reference to Jara. International Research Journal of Pharmacy. 2017;**8**(4):5-8

[29] Towards Long-Term Care Systems in Sub-Saharan Africa: WHO Series on Long-Term Care. Geneva: World Health Organization; 2017 www.who.int License: CCBY-NC-SA.3.0190. assessed October 2018

[30] Keller I, Makipaa A, Kalenscher TM, Kalache A. Global Survey on Geriatrics in the Medical Curriculum. Geneva: World Health Organization; 2002 www.who.int assessed October 2018

[31] Vellas B, Morleg JE. Geriatrics in the 21st century. Journal of Nutrition and Healthy Aging. 2018;**22**(2):186-190

[32] Musunuru K, Mallela J. A systematic review on the role of healthcare administration in geriatric care. Open Journal of Geriatric Medicine. 2018;**4**(2):1-3

[33] Nishinaga M. Comprehensive geriatric assessment and team intervention. JMAJ. 2007;**50**(6):461-466

[34] Wilber ST, Gerson LW, Terrel KM, Carpenter CR, Shah MN, Heard K, et al. Geriatric emergency medicine and the 2006 Institute of Medicine reports from the committee on the future of emergency care in the US health system. Academy of. Emergency Medicine. 2006;**13**(12):1345-1351 www.aemj.org assessed October 2018

[35] Fisher JM, Garside M, Hunt K, Lo N. Geriatric medicine workforce planning: A giant geriatric problem or has the tide turned? Clinical Medicine. 2014;**14**(2):1026

[36] World Health Organization. Ageing. www.who.int

[37] Ssensamba JT, Mukuru M, Nakafeero M, Sseryonga R, Kiwanuka SN. Health systems readiness to provide geriatric friendly care services in Uganda: A cross-sectional study. BMC Geriatrics. 2019;**19**:256. DOI: 10.186/s12877-019-1272-2

[38] Assumcao M, Pinto S, Jose H. Public and health policy for the aged in Africa to the south of Saraa. Revista Brasileira de Enfermagem. 2020;**73**(Suppl 3): e20190313. DOI: 101590/0034-7167-2019-0313

[39] Singh S, Bajorek B. Defining elderly in clinical practice guidelines for pharmacotherapy. Pharmacy Practice. 2014;**12**(4):489-490 www.pharmacypractice.org accessed October 2018

[40] Ayokunle AM, Oyeyemi FT, Onipede W, O TF, Olagunju AE, Makinde GB, et al. The definitions and onset of an old person in South-Western Nigeria. Educational Gerontology. 2015;**41**(7):494-503. DOI: 10.1080/03601277.2014.1003492

[41] www.un.org Assessed October 2018

[42] www.who.int Assessed October 2018

[43] Raveendra L. A clinical study of geriatric dermatoses. Our Dermatology Online. 2014;**5**(3):235-239

[44] Sobokta L, Schneider SM, Berner YN, Cederholm T, Krznaric Z, Shenkin A, et al. ESPENN guidelines on parenteral nutrition: Geriatrics. Clinical Nutrition. 2008;**28**:461-466

[45] Adeleke RO, Adebowale TO, Oyinlola O. Profile of elderly patients presented with psychosocial problems in Ibadan. MOJ Gerontology and Geriatrics. 2017;**1**(1):26-36

[46] Abanyam NL. The changing privileges and challenges of older persons in contemporary African society. Global Journal of Art and Human Social Science. 2013;**1**(41):34-43

[47] Asagba A. Research and the formulation and implantation of ageing policy in Africa: The case of Nigeria. British Society of Gerontology. 2005;**16**(2):39-41

[48] Gyasi RM, Phillips DR, Abass K. Social support networks and psychological well-being in community-dwelling older Ghanaians cohorts. International Psychogeriatrics. 2019;**31**(7):1047-1057

[49] The American Geriatric Society. Why Geriatrics as a Career Choice? www.

americangeriatrics.org Assessed October 2018

[50] The Canadian Geriatrics Society. Geriatric Medicine Profile. www.canadiangeriatrics.ca Assessed October 2018

[51] Misha AA. The concept of successful aging. International Journal of Human and Health Sciences. 2017;**01**(01):22-25

[52] Royal College of Physicians and Surgeons of Canada. Objectives of Training in the Subspecialty of Geriatric Medicine. www.royalcollege.ca

[53] Royal College of Physicians of London. The Diploma in Geriatric Medicine. www.rcplondon.ac.uk Assessed October 2018

[54] Adedokun MO. Caring for the elderly: Towards a better community. European Journal of Educational Services. 2010;**2**(3):283-291

[55] Okoye UO. Community-based care for homebound elderly persons in Nigeria. A policy option. International Journal of Innovative Research in Science, Engineering and Technology. 2013;**2**(12):7086-7091

Section 2

Physical–psychosocial Relationships: Moving towards Healthy Aging

Chapter 4

Does Physical Activity Mediate the Effect of Loneliness on Inflammatory and Metabolic Processes?

Sharon Shiovitz-Ezra, Ohad Parag and Howard Litwin

Abstract

The study to be presented in the chapter explores one potential behavioral mechanism by which loneliness affects inflammatory and metabolic processes in old age. Specifically, it addresses whether physical activity mediates the loneliness—inflammatory/metabolic dysregulation association. Multivariate linear regressions were applied to data derived from the Health and Retirement Study (HRS). The findings revealed that loneliness was prospectively associated with elevated values of log C-reactive protein (log-CRP) and with amplified levels of Glycated hemoglobin (HbA1c), Cystatin C (CysC), and Body Mass Index (BMI), after controlling for socio-demographics. Second, physical activity mediated the association between loneliness with prospective values of log-CRP and also mediated associations between loneliness and prospective levels of metabolic biomarkers. These findings affirm the contribution (i.e., the mediation), of physical activity to the associations between loneliness and immune and metabolic processes and provide insights concerning the mechanism by which this social—biological connection operates.

Keywords: bio-markers, inflammation, metabolic dysregulation, HRS, physical activity, metabolic processes

1. Introduction

A sense of loneliness is a subjective marker for deficits in one's social relationships conceptualized as the discrepancy between the self-perceived extent of contact and support desired and the actual level of contact and support received [1]. This disparity leads to a cascade of behavioral, neural, hormonal, cellular, and molecular changes in the short-term [2]. In the longer-term, loneliness has been shown to negatively affect health and diminish longevity, especially among older adults [3, 4].

Because of the advancement of the study of the association that exists between loneliness and health in old age, interest has been fostered in better understanding the possible biological basis of this relationship. This is especially the case in industrialized countries where population aging is dramatically increasing and, correspondingly, the costs of dealing with poor health in old age are escalating [5]. Chronic inflammation is one of the postulated bio-physiological pathways through which loneliness may exacerbate the poor health of many older adults. Findings show, for example, that inflammatory responses that lead to prolonged and systemic immune responses, such as a rise in C-reactive protein (CRP) levels, are correlated with feelings of loneliness [6], while these same inflammatory responses also predict cardiovascular diseases [7] and higher mortality [8].

Another possible explanation for the association between loneliness and health in late life is that metabolic dysregulation serves as a trajectory in which different aspects of social disconnectedness, especially loneliness, are associated with the health condition. Studies underscore that loneliness predicts metabolic dysregulation as indicated by high systolic blood pressure and age-related differences in metabolic functioning [9], on the one hand, and that metabolic processes are linked to one's health state, on the other hand. An example of the latter case is that levels of Glycated hemoglobin (Hba1c), a glucose concentration measure, serve as criteria for diabetes diagnosis [10]. In addition, Body Mass Index (BMI), a measure to assess obesity, as well as Cystatin C, (CysC), a biomarker of kidney function, both prospectively predict cardiovascular events and all-cause mortality among older adults [11, 12]. Recently, loneliness was found to be associated with a change for the worse in several metabolic bio-markers. Specifically, lonely older adults had 39–71% higher odds of developing prospective risk levels in HbA1c, BMI, and metabolic burden [13].

The mechanism through which loneliness is related to inflammatory and metabolic markers, respectively, is yet to be elucidated. Hawkley and Cacioppo [14] outlined several potential mechanisms by which loneliness affects health including compromising health behaviors. They argued that the lonely individual perceives the social world as threatening and that this perspective weakens his or her self-regulation, thus creating patterns of health-compromising behaviors such as physical inactivity, which cause a deterioration of health [14–16]. This hypothesis was supported by Segrin & Passalacqua [17] who found that exercise mediated the association of loneliness with self-rated health. More recently another cross-sectional study carried out in Denmark found that physical inactivity mediated the relationship between loneliness and adverse health condition such as cardiovascular disease [18].

However, to the best of our knowledge, the role of physical activity as a significant agent in the prospective association between loneliness and inflammatory and metabolic biomarkers has not yet been fully tested within the same study. Studies substantiated the relationship between loneliness and engagement in physical activity, with loneliness found to be associated with transitioning from physically active status to sedentary status [19], on one hand. Studies report a positive association between physical activity and improvement in inflammatory and metabolic regulation, as manifested by a more substantial reduction in CRP levels [20] and by higher HbA1c declines [21], on the other hand.

Consequently, the aim of the current inquiry is to address the dynamics of this assumed relationship systematically. Toward this end, we examine whether physical activity mediates the postulated association between loneliness and two key biological processes among older adults, looking specifically at its effect in relation to both inflammation and metabolic deficits. The focus on older adults in the current study is warranted insofar as research has validated that older people face loneliness more frequently [22]. They are also more prone to immune and metabolic defectiveness than are younger adults [23, 24]. Moreover, social-physiological interconnections have more prominent effects on older age cohorts [9]. The spotlight on the older age strata is also crucial in that previous studies have revealed that loneliness accelerates physiological aging [16].

2. Materials and methods

2.1 Data

The data for the analysis were drawn from the Health and Retirement Study (HRS), a nationally representative, a biennial longitudinal survey sponsored by the National Institute on Aging and the Social Security Administration, and run by the Survey Research Center at the University of Michigan's Institute for Social Research. The HRS gathers a wide range of economic, social, and health data on older adults [25]. The Institutional Review Board of the University of Michigan granted ethical approval [26]. The loneliness data and all of the social-demographic variables for the present inquiry were retrieved from Wave 7 (2006) of the HRS. Information on the frequency of physical activity was taken from Wave 8 (2008). The blood-based inflammatory and metabolic markers, which served as the outcome measures in the current analysis were collected in Wave 9 (2010) of the survey (The HRS collects biomeasures from a portion of the respondents at each Wave, on a rotation basis, and not from the entire sample [27]). The BMI scores, another metabolic outcome, were also taken from the Wave 9 data.

We limited the analytic sample to respondents aged 60 and above who had valid data regarding social-demographic background, loneliness, frequency of physical activity, and at least one inflammatory or metabolic bio-marker from Wave 9. The resultant analytic sample thus numbered some 3,735 respondents. This number varied slightly across the respective multivariate analyses, as has been similarly reported in related studies [28]. Descriptive statistics of the respondents in the current study are reported in **Table 1**.

	Wave 7	Wave 9
Women	58.4%	
Age, mean (SD)	71.1 (7.2)	
White	84.3%	
Married	66.9%	
>12 years of education	25.7%	
Currently working	14.3%	
Depressed	10.7%	
Loneliness, mean (SE)	4.3 (0.03)	
Moderate physical activity, at least once a week (wave 8)	54.1%	
Log-CRP, mg/dL, mean (SE)		0.16 (0.01)
Hba1c, %, mean (SE)		5.87 (0.02)
BMI, kg/m2, mean (SE)		29.77 (0.11)
CysC, mean (SE)		1.22 (0.01)

Table 1.
Demographics, loneliness scores, frequency of physical activity, and bio- markers values of the sample.

2.2 Variables

2.2.1 Predictor

Loneliness was evaluated by the abbreviated 3-item form of the R-UCLA Loneliness Scale, a widely used questionnaire that was developed for use in large-scale surveys and was proven to be valid and reliable [29]. Participants were asked on a 3-point scale, ranging from 1 (hardly ever) to 3 (often), how often they felt a sense of (1) being left out, (2) lack of companionship, and (3) isolation. The three items were summed to create a scale score ranging from 3 to 9, with higher scores representing a greater extent of loneliness. As can be seen in **Table 1**, the average loneliness score was M = 4.3, with SE = 0.03.

2.2.2 Outcomes—Bio-measures

The bio-measures (except for BMI) were produced through the collection of Dried Blood Spot (DBS) samples, a minimally invasive and highly valid method [30]. Inflammatory processes were marked by values of CRP, subsequently log-transformed due to skewed distributions, as has been done previously [31]. Respondents with CRP levels >10 mg/L were excluded from the current CRP analyses because we were interested in low-grade inflammation, also in accordance with Yang et al. [31]. Metabolic processes were represented by levels of –Hba1c, [10] and Cystatin C (CysC, [32]), as well as by BMI (weight/height^2) [33].

2.2.3 Mediator

Respondents were asked about the frequency of moderate physical activity that they carry out in their daily life ("How often do you take part in sports or activities that are moderately energetic such as gardening, cleaning the car, walking at a moderate pace"). Vigorous physical activity ("How often do you take part in sports or activities that are vigorous, such as running or jogging, swimming, cycling, aerobics or gym workout, tennis, or digging with a spade or shove") was also explored for sensitivity analysis. Responses for both types of activities (moderate/vigorous) ranged in the current analysis from 1 ("hardly ever or never") to 5 ("every day").

2.2.4 Covariates

Variables that have been shown in other analyses to be relevant to the association that exists between social network relationships and levels of inflammatory and metabolic bio-measures among middle-aged and older adults served as covariates in the current inquiry [6, 31, 34]. Specifically, the regressions were adjusted by gender (men, women), age (60–96), ethnic affiliation (White, Black, or Hispanic), marital status (married, not married), the extent of formal education (up to and including a high-school diploma/GED, more than a high-school diploma/GED), employment status (working/not working) and depression (Yes/ No). Covariates were gathered in Wave 7, aside from depression, which was measured at Wave 8, due to low response rate on this question at Wave 7. The reference categories were men, white, not married, up to and including a high-school diploma/GED, currently not working and not depressed.

2.3 Data analysis

Multiple multivariate linear procedures were employed. The main effect of loneliness on the four bio-markers was analyzed separately for each of the biomarkers: log CRP, Hba1c, BMI, and CysC, after adjusting for the sundry controls (gender, age, ethnic pertaining, education, marital status, employment status, and depression status). The Ns for the respective analyses were: log-CRP (n = 3127), Hba1c (n = 3402), BMI (n = 3538), CysC (n = 3362). The STATA software program 15.0 was used in this stage of the study.

In the second phase of the analysis, physical activity was added to the regressions as a mediator. However, this potential mediation effect was explored only when the main effect of loneliness was significant in phase 1. The second phase was carried out using the PROCESS macro in the SPSS statistical program. The SPSS analytic software was preferred here because it computes the direct and indirect effects in multiple mediator models, by calculating the product of coefficients [35]. Finally, the significance of the mediation was tested by means of bootstrapping, a nonparametric technique that does not require a-priori assumptions about the data distribution [36]. This method empirically estimates the sampling distribution by repeatedly resampling the data. When the confidence interval of 95 percent, which is based upon 1000 bootstrap samples, excludes zero, the mediation effect is significant [37].

3. Results

3.1 Phase 1: main effects

The Prediction model results showed that being lonely at Wave 7 was associated with having higher log-CRP levels ($\beta = 0.06$, $p < 0.01$), higher Hba1c levels ($\beta = 0.05$, $p < 0.01$), higher BMI scores ($\beta = 0.06$, $p < 0.01$) and higher CysC values ($\beta = 0.05$, $p < 0.01$) at Wave 9, after adjusting for gender, age, ethnic pertaining, education, marital status, employment status and depression status.

3.2 Phase 2: mediation effect

The Prediction models in **Figures 1–4**, depict the associations of loneliness with prospective levels of log-CRP, Hba1c, BMI, and CysC with physical activity as a potential mediator. We elaborate here on the association between loneliness with prospective levels of log-CRP (**Figure 1**) since all other associations present a similar pattern of results. As demonstrated in **Figure 1**, higher levels of loneliness were significantly associated with increased prospective values of log-CRP (path c). However, the beta coefficient for the effect of loneliness on the frequency of physical activity (path a) and the beta coefficient for the effect of frequency of physical activity on levels of log-CRP (path b), were both significant. Also, the direct effect of loneliness in the presence of the mediator (path c') was weaker than the total effect of loneliness (path c). This highlights a feasible indirect effect of loneliness through the frequency of physical activity [38]. In other words, greater loneliness decreased the frequency of subsequent physical exercise ($\beta = -0.14$) and this reduction in physical activity elevated the prospective levels of log-CRP ($\beta = -0.11$). When the mediator was used, the direct effect between loneliness and Log-CRP levels was still significant but weaker, which suggests partial mediation.

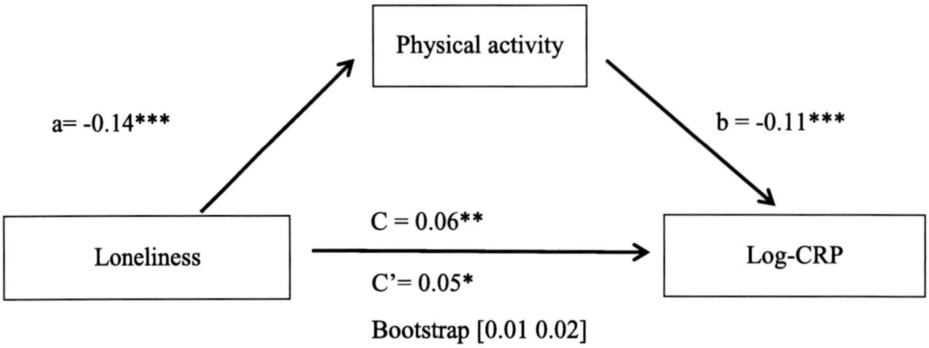

Figure 1.
The mediation effect of physical activity upon the association of loneliness with prospective log-CRP levels. Adjusted by all variables in the Prediction model. Based upon 1000 bootstrap samples.

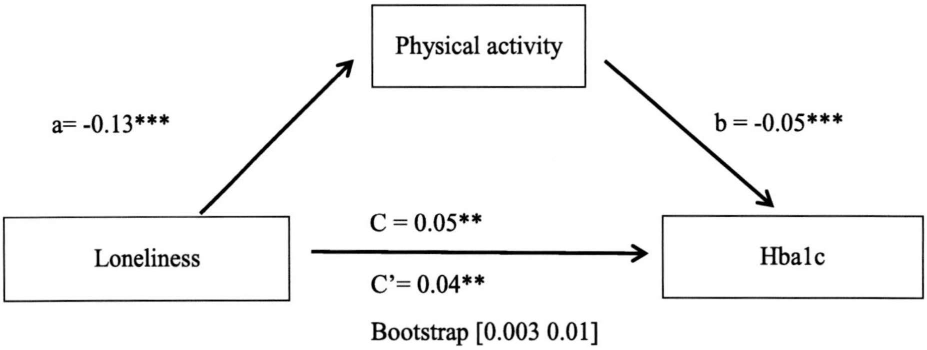

Figure 2.
The mediation effect of physical activity upon the association of loneliness with prospective Hba1c levels. Adjusted by all variables in the Prediction model. Based upon 1000 bootstrap samples.

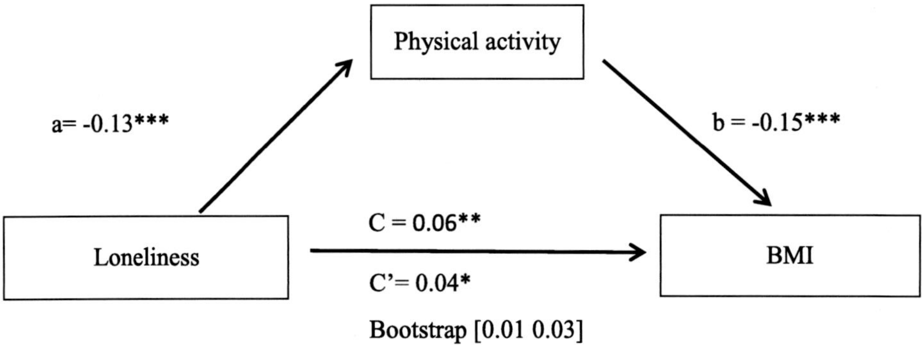

Figure 3.
The mediation effect of physical activity upon the association of loneliness with prospective BMI levels. Adjusted by all variables in the prediction model. Based upon 1000 bootstrap samples.

To test whether the mediation effect was significant we applied a bootstrap method. As may be seen in **Figure 1**, the association between loneliness with prospective levels of log-CRP was partially mediated because path c' was still significant. The confidence interval of 95 percent, which was based upon 1000 bootstrap samples, was between 0.01 and 0.02, thus indicating mediation [37]. As already mentioned,

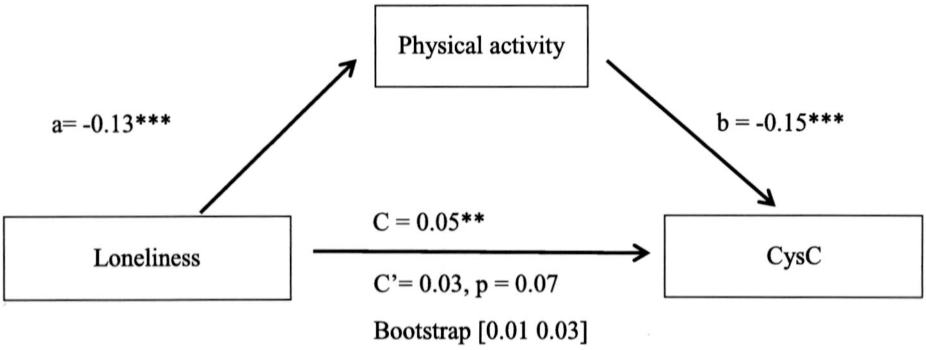

Figure 4.
The mediation effect of physical activity upon the association of loneliness with prospective CysC levels. Adjusted by all variables in the prediction model. Based upon 1000 bootstrap samples.

similar results emerged in all the other relevant associations that were found to be significant in the first phase (i.e, between loneliness and the prospective concentrations of metabolic biomarkers (**Figures 2–4**).

Dividing the (standardized) indirect effect by the (standardized) total effect [39] showed that the indirect path of physical activity accounted for 25 percent of the association of loneliness with prospective values of log-CRP, 14 percent of the association with Hba1c, 32 percent of the association with BMI, and 36 percent of the association with CysC (not shown in the Figures). Sensitivity analysis of engagement in more vigorous physical activity showed very similar results (not shown).

4. Discussion

This study examined whether physical activity mediates the effect of loneliness on inflammatory and metabolic processes among older Americans. We found, in the first phase of the study, that loneliness was, indeed, associated with increased levels of inflammation, measured 4 years later, as reflected by heightened values of (log) CRP [6]. Similarly, loneliness was associated with subsequent low metabolic regulation, also measured 4 years later, as manifested by elevated concentrations in all three of the metabolic measures that were examined: BMI, Hba1c, and CysC. These measures encompass several different aspects of metabolic processes, such as glucose concentration, kidney function, and CVD profiling, thus emphasizing the effect of loneliness on metabolic process as a whole [10, 33].

As noted, the primary focus of the current study was to consider whether physical activity mediates the loneliness—biomarker associations that emerged in the initial phase of the analysis. The findings show that the association of loneliness with the inflammatory marker log-CRP was partially mediated by the physical activity indirect pathway, which accounted for a quarter of the total effect. In addition, all of the significant associations between loneliness and prospective metabolic bio-markers were either partially or entirely mediated by physical activity. Of particular note is that this indirect effect was not at all minor, as it accounted for a substantial portion of the associations between loneliness and prospective BMI and CysC levels, with about a third of these associations being attributed to it. To the best of our knowledge, these findings are the first to affirm the contribution (i.e., the mediation), of physical activity to the associations between loneliness and immune and metabolic processes and to provide insights concerning the mechanism by which this social—biological connection operates.

The results of this study have important implications insofar as they suggest the deleterious effects of loneliness upon inflammatory and metabolic processes in later life, which have been reported in prior studies [6, 7, 9], can be mediated by physical activity. Our analyses showed that this might indeed occur due to engagement in any level of physical activity, whether moderate or vigorous. This implies that even moderate physical activity serves as a mechanism by which loneliness affects health in old age.

One potential limitation should be taken into account when interpreting the results of our analysis. We do not control whether the loneliness scores that were taken as the baseline indicator in the current analysis (Wave 7 of the HRS) represent transient or chronic loneliness. These two types of loneliness are conceptually different. Whereas transient loneliness may motivate individuals to reconnect with other individuals, loneliness that is accrued over time increases withdrawal [15]. This is a minor shortcoming; however, insofar as most older people have stable loneliness ratings over time [40].

In conclusion, this study identifies an important psycho-physiological mechanism that may be present among older adults. It documents that physical activity mediates the effect of loneliness on inflammatory and metabolic processes in a representative national sample of older Americans. Reduced engagement in physical activities in later life explains to some degree the deleterious health effects of loneliness.

Acknowledgements

The HRS (Health and Retirement Study) is sponsored by the National Institute on Aging (grant number NIA U01AG009740) and is conducted by the University of Michigan.

Author details

Sharon Shiovitz-Ezra[1*], Ohad Parag[2] and Howard Litwin[2]

1 Paul Baerwald School of Social Work and Social Welfare, The Hebrew University of Jerusalem, Jerusalem, Israel

2 Israel Gerontological Data Center (IGDC), The Hebrew University of Jerusalem, Jerusalem, Israel

*Address all correspondence to: sharon.shiovitz@mail.huji.ac.il

References

[1] Peplau LA, Perlman D. Perspectives on loneliness. In: Peplau LA, Perlman D, editors. Loneliness: A Sourcebook of Current Theory, Research and Therapy. New York: Wiley; 1982. pp. 1-8

[2] Cacioppo JT, Cacioppo S. Loneliness in the modern age: An evolutionary theory of loneliness (ETL). Advances in Experimental Social Psychology. 2018;**58**:127-197

[3] Jessen MAB, Pallesen AVJ, Kriegbaum M, Kristiansen M. The association between loneliness and health–a survey-based study among middle-aged and older adults in Denmark. Aging & Mental Health. 2017;**22**(10): 1338-1343

[4] Luo Y, Hawkley LC, Waite LJ, Cacioppo JT. Loneliness, health, and mortality in old age: A national longitudinal study. Social Science & Medicine. 2012;**74**(6):907-914

[5] Cacioppo JT, Cacioppo S. Social relationships and health: The toxic effects of perceived social isolation. Social and Personality Psychology Compass. 2014;**8**(2):58-72

[6] Steptoe A, Owen N, Kunz-Ebrecht SR, Brydon L. Loneliness and neuroendocrine, cardiovascular, and inflammatory stress responses in middle-aged men and women. Psychoneuroendocrinology. 2004;**29**(5):593-611

[7] Honda H, Qureshi AR, Heimbürger O, Barany P, Wang K, Pecoits-Filho R, et al. Serum albumin, C-reactive protein, interleukin 6, and fetuin a as predictors of malnutrition, cardiovascular disease, and mortality in patients with ESRD. American Journal of Kidney Diseases. 2006;**47**(1):139-148

[8] Yeun JY, Levine RA, Mantadilok V, Kaysen GA. C-reactive protein predicts all-cause and cardiovascular mortality in hemodialysis patients. American Journal of Kidney Diseases. 2000;**35**(3):469-476

[9] Hawkley LC, Masi CM, Berry JD, Cacioppo JT. Loneliness is a unique predictor of age-related differences in systolic blood pressure. Psychology and Aging. 2006;**21**(1):152-164

[10] American Diabetes Association. Standards of medical care in diabetes–2010. Diabetes Care. 2010;**33**(Suppl. 1):S11-S61

[11] Asia Pacific Cohort Studies Collaboration. Body mass index and cardiovascular disease in the Asia-Pacific Region: An overview of 33 cohorts involving 310 000 participants. International Journal of Epidemiology. 2004;**33**(41):751-758

[12] Shlipak MG, Sarnak MJ, Katz R, Fried LF, Seliger SL, Newman AB, et al. Cystatin C and the risk of death and cardiovascular events among elderly persons. New England Journal of Medicine. 2005;**352**(20):2049-2060

[13] Shiovitz-Ezra S, Parag O. Does loneliness 'get under the skin'? Associations of loneliness with subsequent change in inflammatory and metabolic markers. Aging & Mental Health. 2018;**2018**:1-9

[14] Hawkley LC, Cacioppo JT. Loneliness matters: A theoretical and empirical review of consequences and mechanisms. Annals of Behavioral Medicine. 2010;**40**(2):218-227

[15] Cacioppo JT, Hawkley LC. Perceived social isolation and cognition.

Trends in Cognitive Sciences. 2009;**13**(10):447-454

[16] Hawkley LC, Cacioppo JT. Aging and loneliness: Downhill quickly? Current Directions in Psychological Science. 2007;**16**(4):187-191

[17] Segrin C, Passalacqua SA. Functions of loneliness, social support, health behaviors, and stress in association with poor health. Health Communication. 2010;**25**(4):312-322

[18] Christiansen J, Larsen FB, Lasgaard M. Do stress, health behavior, and sleep mediate the association between loneliness and adverse health conditions among older people? Social Science & Medicine. 2016;**152**:80-86

[19] Hawkley LC, Thisted RA, Cacioppo JT. Loneliness predicts reduced physical activity: Cross sectional & longitudinal analyses. Health Psychology. 2009;**28**(3):354-363

[20] Albert MA, Glynn RJ, Ridker PM. Effect of physical activity on serum C-reactive protein. The American Journal of Cardiology. 2004;**93**(2):221-225

[21] Umpierre D, Ribeiro PA, Kramer CK, Leitão CB, Zucatti AT, Azevedo MJ, et al. Physical activity advice only or structured exercise training and association with HbA1c levels in type 2 diabetes: A systematic review and meta-analysis. JAMA. 2011;**305**(17):1790-1799

[22] Tijhuis MA, De Jong-Gierveld J, Feskens EJ, Kromhout D. Changes in and factors related to loneliness in older men. The Zutphen Elderly Study. Age and Ageing. 1999;**28**(5):491-495

[23] Ershler WB, Keller ET. Age-associated increased interleukin-6 gene expression, late-life diseases, and frailty. Annual Review of Medicine. 2000;**51**(1):245-270

[24] Ford ES, Giles WH, Dietz WH. Prevalence of the metabolic syndrome among US adults: Findings from the third National Health and Nutrition Examination Survey. JAMA. 2002;**287**(3): 356-359

[25] Heisler M, Cole I, Weir D, Kerr EA, Hayward RA. Does physician communication influence older patients' diabetes self-management and glycemic control? Results from the Health and Retirement Study (HRS). The Journals of Gerontology Series A: Biological Sciences and Medical Sciences. 2007;**62**(12):1435-1442

[26] World Medical Association. Ethical principles for medical research involving human subjects. Bulletin of the World Health Organization. 2001;**79**(4):37

[27] Mitchell UA, Ailshire JA, & Crimmins EM. Change in cardiometabolic risk among blacks, whites, and hispanics: Findings from the Health and Retirement Study. The Journals of Gerontology: Series A. 2018;**74**(2):240-246

[28] Assari S. Association between obesity and depression among American Blacks: Role of ethnicity and gender. Journal of Racial and Ethnic Health Disparities. 2014;**1**(1):36-44

[29] Hughes ME, Waite LJ, Hawkley LC, Cacioppo JT. short scale for measuring loneliness in large surveys: Results from two population-based studies. Research on Aging. 2004;**26**(6):655-672

[30] McDade TW, Williams S, Snodgrass JJ. What a drop can do: Dried blood spots as a minimally invasive method for integrating biomarkers into population-based research. Demography. 2007;**44**(4):899-925

[31] Yang YC, Boen C, Gerken K, Li T, Schorpp K, Harris KM. Social relationships and physiological

determinants of longevity across the human life span. Proceedings of the National Academy of Sciences. 2016;**113**(3):578-583

[32] Laterza OF, Price CP, Scott MG. Cystatin C: An improved estimator of glomerular filtration rate? Clinical Chemistry. 2002;**48**(5):699-707

[33] Katzmarzyk PT, Srinivasan SR, Chen W, Malina RM, Bouchard C, Berenson GS. Body mass index, waist circumference, and clustering of cardiovascular disease risk factors in a biracial sample of children and adolescents. Pediatrics. 2004;**114**(2):e198-e205

[34] Hawkley LC, Hughes ME, Waite LJ, Masi CM, Thisted RA, Cacioppo JT. From social structural factors to perceptions of relationship quality and loneliness: The Chicago health, aging, and social relations study. The Journals of Gerontology Series B: Psychological Sciences and Social Sciences. 2008;**63**(6):S375-S384

[35] Hayes AF. Introduction to Mediation, Moderation, and Conditional Process Analysis: A Regression-based Approach. New York, NY: Guilford Press; 2013

[36] Preacher KJ, Hayes AF. Asymptotic and resampling strategies for assessing and comparing indirect effects in multiple mediator models. Behavior Research Methods. 2008;**40**(3):879-891

[37] Preacher KJ, Hayes AF. SPSS and SAS procedures for estimating indirect effects in simple mediation models. Behavior Research Methods. 2004;**36**(4):717-731

[38] Baron RM, Kenny DA. The moderator–mediator variable distinction in social psychological research: Conceptual, strategic, and statistical considerations. Journal of Personality and Social Psychology. 1986;**51**(6):1173

[39] Preacher KJ, Kelley K. Effect size measures for mediation models: Quantitative strategies for communicating indirect effects. Psychological Methods. 2011;**16**(2):93

[40] Victor CR, Bowling A. A longitudinal analysis of loneliness among older people in Great Britain. The Journal of psychology. 2012;**146**(3):313-331

Chapter 5

Perspective Chapter: Social Distancing and Isolation – Unintended Consequences, Concerns, and Antidotes for Older Adults

Amy Joy Lanou, Jeff Jones, Louise Noble, Thomas Smythe, Lauren Alexa Gambrill, Emma Olson and Tasha Woodall

Abstract

Social isolation and loneliness are critical social drivers of health and need to be recognized as such. Safety efforts due to the COVID-19 pandemic have increased social isolation, highlighted the digital divide for older adults and rural communities, and have exacerbated related health concerns especially among older adults. Opportunities for increasing social connectedness of older adults and others who are isolated must be prioritized to decrease the impact of social isolation and loneliness on mental and physical health. Recommendations for policies, programs, and other actions addressing social isolation as a determinant of healthy aging by supporting community and individual social connectedness are highlighted using case examples from the western region of North Carolina. The purpose of this chapter is to urge policy makers and health professionals to prioritize policies, programs, and support for social connectedness as an antidote to turn the tide on the widespread impact of social isolation on the health of older adults.

Keywords: social isolation, loneliness, social distancing, social connection, older adults

1. Introduction

Although definitions vary, loneliness is most often described as a subjective term referring to the discrepancy between the quantity and quality of relationships that one has and what they desire. Social isolation, a more objective measure, has been alternatively defined as the "state of having few social relationships or infrequent social contact with others" or the "pervasive lack of social contact or communication, participation in social activities or having a confidant" among others [1, 2].

A growing body of evidence indicates that social isolation and loneliness are impacting health and health outcomes around the world. Two international literature reviews recently completed in the United Kingdom and in Finland included findings from studies in 23 countries across five continents. The Centre of Excellence for Public Health at Queen's University in Northern Ireland reviewed social isolation interventions in 33 studies conducted in 21 countries, and concluded that tailored approaches are needed to address loneliness and social isolation [3]. Tampere University in Finland reviewed 23 studies conducted in 13 countries and found that technological approaches are useful for assessing loneliness and social isolation among older adults and for alleviating loneliness safely without risk of infection transmission due to in person contact [4]. Both reviews found that the amount of research from the international scientific community on this topic has increased significantly during the past decade [3, 4].

Social isolation prevalence varies worldwide, but reports indicate rates as high as a third of older adults aged 65+ in some countries. Rates in European countries range from 19.6–34% and in Latin America from 25.3% to 32.4% [5]. A National Academy of Medicine (NAM) Consensus Study (2020) reported a 24% rate of social isolation in the U.S., while prevalence rates in Australia and India were lower at 19% and 18.3%, respectively [6]. The association between social isolation and loneliness is complex. Rates of loneliness are lower than rates of social isolation in some countries but exceed them in others. The NAM study ("Social Isolation and Loneliness in Older Adults: Opportunities for the Health Care System") reported that 43% of adults aged 60+ in the U.S. report feeling lonely, while rates in Europe are much lower and range from 3–10% [7, 8].

The NAM report also noted that social isolation is associated with a 50% increased risk of dementia, 29% increased risk of heart disease and 32% increased risk of stroke, and others have found that social isolation presents a substantial risk for increased morbidity, premature mortality and dysregulation of health biomarkers (blood pressure, C-reactive protein and cortisol levels) comparable to the risk associated with obesity, hypertension or daily tobacco use and is also associated with mental health morbidities such as depression, anxiety and dementia [9–11]. Loneliness is "characterized by impairments in attention, cognition, affect, and behavior that take a toll on morbidity and mortality through their impact on genetic, neural and hormonal mechanisms" [10]. It is associated with higher rates of depression, anxiety and suicide and, among heart failure patients, is associated with a nearly 4-fold increased risk of death, 68% increased risk of hospitalization, and 57% increased risk of emergency department visits [6].

The digital divide may further compound the risk of social isolation for older adults. Although technology use in this population increased 55% from 2000 to 2016, one third of older adults report never using the internet, and rates of smartphone ownership in adults aged 65+ remain 42% lower than that of adults aged 18 to 64. This same study found especially low rates of access and use among adults aged 80+. Adults aged 65 to 69 are about twice as likely to say they ever go online (82% vs. 44%) or have broadband at home (66% vs. 28%) and roughly four times as likely to say they own smartphones (59% vs. 17%) as their counterparts aged 80+ [12]. In addition to access and technology usage issues, hearing loss and impaired vision, common in the older adult population, can further complicate digital service accessibility [13]. Shteinlukht found that 60% of older adult respondents reported challenges utilizing digital platforms for virtual appointments [14].

This excess burden of vulnerability and disparate use of technology is further compounded by challenges unique to rural areas. The Western North Carolina (WNC) region has a 44% higher proportion of persons age 65+ than North Carolina as a whole and, of the 23 counties in the region, 83% [15] are classified as rural [16, 17]. Henning-Smith found that "older adults in rural areas were more than 10 percentage points more likely to report feeling left out often or at least some of the time," and 5% of them reported having no friends at all [18]. Another Henning-Smith study (2020) found that, "although older adults in rural areas report having larger social networks than their urban area counterparts, they also report higher levels of loneliness, indicating structural barriers to connecting" [19]. The disproportionate impact of the digital divide on older adults in rural areas has also been well documented. A Pew Research Center report demonstrated consistently lower rates of smartphone, computer and tablet ownership and lower rates of access to broadband internet at home in rural adults vs. urban adults (two-thirds vs. three-quarters) [15]. Rural adults who do have internet access are often unable to participate in synchronous activities such as video-conferencing for telehealth or social calls due to slower speeds and poor, unstable connectivity caused by low bandwidth [20]. Even those who have internet access and use it for social contact may not fully benefit, as several studies have demonstrated that indirect modes of contact such as Facebook and other internet-based platforms may not influence health in the same way or to the same degree as direct, in-person contact [21]. "As a result, older adults in rural areas are among the most likely to be left out of any creative, technologically-based adaptations to meet social and other needs during this crisis" [22].

Social isolation and loneliness impact health at the individual level and, arguably, also at the social or "conditions" level. The World Health Organization (WHO) defines social determinants of health as "the non-medical factors that influence health outcomes" or "the conditions in which people are born, grow, work, live, and age, and the wider set of forces and systems shaping the conditions of daily life." While some lists of social determinants of health include social isolation or connectedness, as in WHO's list with "social inclusion and non-discrimination," often the factors shaping this condition of daily life are left out of efforts to address social determinants of health [23]. Place is an important factor that shapes conditions of daily life [23]. For example, living in a rural, mountainous, or otherwise remote region makes social connection, broadband access, and health care utilization more difficult. Other forces and systems at play include social norms and social policies such as those implemented to curb the spread of COVID-19 infection which concomitantly increased social isolation across the globe.

In this chapter, the unintended consequences of measures to reduce COVID-19 morbidity and mortality on social isolation are outlined, followed by a discussion of the importance of supporting and re-engaging social connectedness to combat social isolation, and recommendations to policy makers, communities and health professionals on how to effectively respond to these concerns are discussed. Considering social isolation as a social determinant of health and taking action to increase social connectedness among is important to reduce chronic disease, and improve physical and mental well-being for older adults.

2. Impact of pandemic mitigation on older adults in the United States

On March 13, 2020, as a result of the COVID-19 pandemic, the President of the United States declared a national emergency [24]. At the same time, the majority of US states issued stay-at-home orders in response to the pandemic [25]. By April of 2020, the White House Coronavirus Taskforce and the Centers for Disease Control (CDC) were recommending that individuals wear face coverings to slow the spread of SARS-CoV-2 [26]. In many US states, face coverings were eventually mandated in public areas, and various social distancing policies persisted well into the pandemic [27].

These measures ultimately mitigated viral transmission and concomitant harms in the US [28, 29]. Nevertheless, many unmistakable harms are inherent to pandemic mitigation efforts as well [2, 30]. The potential for harm is especially concerning for the older adult population. In an attempt to shield vulnerable populations from severe illness and death, policymakers and health officials also risked raising their susceptibility to the deleterious physiological, psychological, and emotional effects of social isolation.

In comparison with 18–29-year-old individuals, 67–74-year-olds are five times more likely to be hospitalized for COVID-19 and 65 times more likely to die from the disease. For those 75–84 years old, hospitalization is 8 times more likely, while death is 150 times more likely than for young adults. For people who have reached 85+ years of age, hospitalizations are 10 times more likely, and they are 370 times more likely to die of COVID-19 [31]. In March 2020, older adults also reported that they perceived their risk of death to be higher than that of younger adults or children [32]. Taken together, older adults are right to feel heightened concern about the potential consequences of contracting SARS-CoV-2. And now, even in light of the availability and utilization of effective vaccinations, heightened fear of contracting the virus lingers among some older adults [33].

The authors have heard stories from community members indicating they were fearful of and avoiding seeking medical care, shopping for essential items, visiting friends and loved ones, receiving gifts, coming in close contact with neighbors, and other activities. At a mass vaccination site in Western North Carolina during the first weeks of vaccine availability, several older adults shared that they had literally not left their homes in a year. Evidence is emerging that this problem is not unique to this region: older adults throughout the US have experienced similar difficulties and were leaving their homes less often [34, 35]. Many put off routine medical care or discontinued health-supporting behaviors such as daily visits to a facility for safe exercise or were no longer able to congregate for shared meals at senior centers, churches or other community gathering sites. An 88-year-old community member visited the Silver Sneakers program at a nearby YMCA 5 to 6 days a week before the "lockdown" and counted on these daily visits for maintaining strength, balance, life outlook and mental acuity. A year and a half into the pandemic he fell at home, broke his hip, and spent 6 weeks hospitalized and in rehabilitation. Six months later, his struggle to regain this strength and baseline level of independence continues. This person's story provides a clear example of how these trends are a cause for concern, not only for ethical reasons but also with respect to health promotion, chronic disease management, and prevention.

While the implementation of shelter-in-place orders, the closing of public spaces, and a decrease in a variety of available services were necessary precautions to slow the spread of the virus, they created a harmful impact on mental health. These policies, in conjunction with advice from the CDC that older adults practice especially rigorous social distancing, have had a large negative impact on the mental health of those 65 and older [36]. While there is reason to believe social isolation in older adults has needed attention for some time, with studies from as early as 2012 estimating that up to 40% of older adults may suffer from social isolation at some point the effects of COVID-19 on day-to-day life brought the impact of social isolation into clearer focus [37]. One older adult explained their experience with isolation, "I don't have very many friends here. I only have a few, and they prefer to send texts. I have no family, and my neighbors aren't very friendly, so I basically have no one to talk to." Data from a 2021 National Health and Aging Trends Study suggests a decrease in weekly in-person contact from 61–39% for at-home individuals and a drop from 56–22% for those in residential care [38].

Even people living in shared housing facilities, retirement homes, long-term care facilities, nursing homes and other congregate sites were subjected to restrictions aimed at reducing exposure. Many were required to stay in their rooms or quarters for months at a time. Some older adults reported reductions in the services offered within their community living facility. Maintenance workers were no longer allowed to enter resident apartments for work orders, laundry and cleaning services were reduced, and tenants' overall support and supervision decreased. One person shared with the authors that these conditions had a significant impact on their mental and emotional wellbeing.

The pandemic necessitated a divergence from in-person communal gatherings, such as worship services, congregate meals, special interest group gatherings, graduations, and other events. Instead, some organizations arranged for individuals to "drive-in" or "drive-up" for special events or transitioned to video conference worship, funerals, graduations or even weddings. Others, like senior centers serving a daily meal, increased their capacity to distribute hot meals to older adults at home by rapidly expanding their food delivery services or partnering with organizations such as Meals on Wheels. Meanwhile, access to gatherings vanished for those who do not own transportation or have digital access, are physically unable to drive or use a device, or are fearful of arranging transportation.

The way people shop for groceries, acquire medications from pharmacies and visit their care providers also underwent dramatic changes during the pandemic. Many younger and more affluent individuals have the option to acquire essential supplies via online shopping and/or the use of delivery applications. While home delivery of hot meals, groceries, and other goods has been important for survival, it also comes at a cost. No-contact delivery options, created for safety reasons, have taken even momentary contact with others out of the equation. For example, a hot meal dropped off without contact is far different than sitting around a table to share a meal with others for feelings of connection.

Similarly, the rate of telemedicine usage increased drastically in April of 2020 and remained a critical part of care delivery well into the pandemic. Yet telemedicine was accessed less often by older adults [39, 40]. Older adults are less likely to access the internet, as underscored by the fact that more than half of adults 80+ years of age were not accessing the internet in the years before the pandemic [41]. Further, individuals with medical conditions and those who live in rural areas also access the internet less frequently than healthy individuals living in non-rural areas [42]. As a result, it is likely that medically complex older adults, especially those who live in a rural area, experienced a higher burden than that of their counterparts. Clinicians' abilities to perform remote monitoring that would typically guide clinical decision-making was also limited since, for example, Medicare Part B coverage for blood pressure monitoring devices is inconsistent and difficult to access [43]. Finally, cognitive, and sensory impairments, more prevalent among older people, pose a barrier to providing effective care via video or telephone visit, even among those who are able to access the proper technology to make these visits feasible.

Wearing a facial covering when in public is arguably one of the simplest and least infringing pandemic mitigation tools on offer. For many people, wearing a facial covering creates negligible restrictions on liberty and does not constitute a legitimate risk to their health or wellbeing. For some older adults however, facial coverings present significant challenges, especially for those experiencing decreased hearing ability. Before the beginning of the pandemic, people with decreased hearing ability were facing difficulties communicating in noisy healthcare settings, which can lead to negative clinical outcomes [44]. Facial coverings can reduce the volume and clarity of verbal communications while also obscuring mouth movements and facial expressions, which many people who have difficulty hearing rely upon to compensate [45]. This loss of sensory input can make communication in both clinical and non-clinical environments more difficult and may lead to lower levels of care efficacy and satisfaction while also causing increased feelings of marginalization, higher levels of confusion, and lower overall levels of connectedness. In addition, face coverings present other challenges. They make it more difficult to recognize others and more difficult to read facial expressions. A shared smile or look of concern can make a difference in how a person feels and responds to others. People with asthma, or other respiratory problems sometimes find wearing a mask especially challenging. Finally, those who wear glasses, have a challenge seeing when they fog up due to mask wearing, which can increase risk of falls, reduce driving safety among other concerns.

The elevated health risks that COVID-19 poses for older adults are a significant burden that weighs heavily on a vulnerable population, creating inequities. Importantly, the most underserved and vulnerable older adults stand to suffer the most. In the context of the current pandemic, social distancing guidelines have created nascent barriers to multiple dimensions of wellbeing in older adults. Therefore, the need to address the negative effects of pandemic mitigation policies on this population is a pressing issue of social justice.

3. Social connectedness as an antidote

Social connectedness or connection to others is a factor in maintaining both physical and emotional wellbeing throughout life. Social connection is the experience of feeling close and connected to others, including feeling valued, cared for, and loved. Dr. Brené Brown, a Research Professor of Social Work at the University of Houston, describes it this way: "Connection is the energy that exists between people when they feel seen, heard and valued; when they can give and receive without judgment; and when they derive sustenance and strength from the relationship" [46]. Described as a core human need and fundamental drive, social connection is an important antidote to social isolation [47].

3.1 Relationships

Feeling socially connected is linked to both the quality and quantity of meaningful relationships with others. The first line of social support often comes in the form of either family or peers in a shared dwelling. Whether living with a spouse or other family member or being part of a living community, physical proximity to other adults often provides some level of social connectedness. For many, human touch is an important expression of connection, and simple acts of touch such as hugs or touching a hand or shoulder provide reassurance, warmth, and are expressions of care [48]. Evidence shows that a healthy level of social support improves the chances of maintaining or initiating healthy behaviors and that increased proximity to other adults results in more social support [49].

3.2 Connection to community

Connectedness is important beyond the individual level. Social connectedness at the community level can also confer important benefits for individual health and society at large. Community gathering places play a significant role in promoting social connection within our society, especially for older adults [50]. Churches, senior centers, affinity groups, and other social hubs all provide a space for individuals to seek out community and social interaction. The use of gyms, YMCAs, malls, and parks for exercise not only improves physical health through movement, but also supports brain health and social connection [49, 51]. Opportunities to engage in learning or share expertise, such as that available at the Osher Lifelong Learning Institutes or institutions of higher education, also provide social connection for engaged members. Regular formal or informal gatherings of friends reduce stress and contribute to social connectedness, such as Moas in the Okinawan tradition "to complain, have fun, lend support," or family, such as intergenerational weekend meals [52].

3.3 Aging in place

Social connectedness is recognized as an important factor in building and maintaining age-friendly communities. Age-friendly communities are those that offer community and individual support for aging in place, defined as the ability to continue to live in the environment of one's choice, often at home or in another familiar place. Using a World Cafe forum, researchers sought to understand social connectedness from those approaching retirement and to learn about factors that would keep aging adults in their respective communities as they age. One of the key themes that emerged was "social reciprocity [defined as] giving and receiving to/from one's community," was perceived to be important in promoting social connectedness. Participants also shared the need for both formal and informal avenues for volunteering in their community as a means of feeling socially engaged [53].

Supports for aging in place in the face of physical limitations which also support social connection include home medical care, meal delivery services, home health aides who support activities of daily living, home safety assessments for falls risk, community health worker supports, and home-based primary care, among other in-home services. In addition to home healthcare agencies, geriatric care managers, senior relocation specialists, senior concierge services, and a vast array of technology services represent some of the emerging industries created to support the transition from a paradigm that has long favored institutionalization for older adults whose needs cannot be met at home, toward one promoting aging in place. Supporting older clients' wishes to sustain their level of social connectedness within their home community may enable those accessing these services to stand a greater chance of aging in place successfully.

3.4 Connecting across the miles

Telephones are a tried-and-true method for connecting people who cannot visit as often as they would like to connect. In recent years, technology has vastly changed the ability of individuals to connect with each other across distances great and small. Through instant messaging and phone calling, social connection is available with the press of a button, and with video chatting faces and body language are visible as well.

While this has helped with social interaction for a large number of people, evidence shows there is a disparity for those 65+ in ability to access and use newer technology, especially those that rely on stable internet access [12]. Projects that increase the availability of smartphones and related technologies and support the use of these devices and services with older adults help to address this digital divide [54]. When devices and broadband are readily available, digital communication can be used to mitigate the negative effects of social isolation and loneliness. Increasing evidence demonstrates online presence and communication is linked to lower depression rates and less reported loneliness in older adults [55]. The ability to connect with family members, friends, or specific community forums such as Alzheimer's Association increases one's connectedness even when performed digitally [56].

4. Effective response is needed: recommendations and case examples

Clear, effective responses are needed to address and mitigate the increases in social isolation among older adults that have been exacerbated by pandemic mitigation strategies [22, 57]. This section outlines five key recommendations and examples of policies and projects poised to make or already making a difference in North Carolina that may be used as models or jumping-off points for other creative efforts to address social isolation, increase social connectedness and promote the health of older adults and their ability to safely continue aging in place.

4.1 Recommendation 1: social isolation and its antidote, social connectedness, should be recognized as a social determinant of health and should be a consideration in health policy decisions

Research has shown that social connectedness is a key social determinant of health (SDOH) that applies to individuals across age, ability, access, and area of service. In fact, the "[f]ormer US Surgeon General Vivek Murthy, MD, MBA, describes loneliness as being similar to thirst. It's the body's way of telling a person that it needs something. We need each other..." [22]. Recognizing the importance of social connection at the individual and community levels affords policymakers an opportunity to improve the health of older adults through such actions as including social connection on lists of agency priorities for addressing social determinants of health. These actions stand to bring this concern, of particular importance for older adults and others disproportionately impacted by COVID mitigation policies, to the forefront.

A case in point is the North Carolina Department of Aging and Adult Services, which has partnered with two university-based teams to bring attention to the need for understanding of social isolation, loneliness, and related health risks including depression and suicide among the 16 Area Agencies on Aging in NC. They have partnered with the NC Center for Health and Wellness and a team of researchers in Georgia to develop and provide resources to partners in the aging network in NC through www.healthyagingNC.com.

Healthy Aging NC is a statewide resource center for evidence-based health programs. The site links a network of program providers to participants seeking classes and support for chronic disease self-management including diabetes, arthritis, and heart disease, falls prevention, chronic pain self-management, improving balance, among others. Many of the providers of evidence-based programs nationwide have traditionally relied on in-person delivery of these programs. The Healthy Aging NC team has provided support and training for partners to rapidly move these programs to remote or hybrid formats, recognizing that losing access to the programs not only reduces opportunities for addressing these chronic conditions and challenges, but also increases social isolation [57].

The reach of these programs marketed and supported through Healthy Aging NC has remained strong during the COVID-19 pandemic with 56 falls prevention workshops offered in 2020 (758 enrolled participants and 289 completers), and with 78 workshops offered in 2021 (677 enrolled participants and 450 completers). In remotely-offered Walk with Ease programs for arthritis and joint pain management, the number of participants enrolled increased dramatically from 20 to 29 in 2018–2019 to 680 in 2020 and 149 in 2021 (personal communication). In addition, as part of this effort to increase connectedness, a new section on social engagement programs, a tool for self-assessment of social isolation, and health coaching opportunities which provide support for changing a behavior have been added to the website to increase referrals to these and other programs.

4.2 Recommendation 2: human service organizations, policymakers, governmental and private foundation funders should prioritize programmatic opportunities to increase social connection for older adults

The onset and continuation of the COVID-19 pandemic has provided opportunities for a wide range of public health, health promotion and human services providers to get creative with reaching socially-isolated adults with readily available technologies. A case example of a program that was rapidly developed to respond to increased social isolation among older adults in WNC is the Social Bridging Project (SBP).

The SBP was implemented as a response to concerns about the potential impact of social isolation on older adults as a result of the pandemic. It was formed as a partnership between the Mountain Area Health Education Center's Center for Health Aging and the NC Center for Health and Wellness at University of North Carolina Asheville with COVID-response funding from the NC Policy Collaboratory. The project's aim is to provide older adults who were isolated or lonely with a source of social connection, technology support and referrals to needed resources. SBP engaged university students as wellness callers to contact older adults in western NC whose lives were impacted by the stay-at-home measures.

During an evaluation of SBP in 2021, several participants remarked upon the impact and consequences of social isolation, including feelings of loneliness, a lack of connectedness or belonging and feelings of 'invisibility' or that their lives did not matter. One participant related, "I don't talk about my feelings very much, even with my children, because I don't want to worry them." Another shared, "ihere's a lot of older people where the children are in other states or other countries, and they're just not available and we forget that we need to be a community. Now that I've lost my vision and can't be on Facebook, I can't stay in touch with my family anymore." Another said, "it's hard when you feel like nobody cares" [58].

The Social Bridging Project team has been making wellness check-in calls to older adults to provide regular social support to isolated older adults in order to mitigate the onset of social isolation and loneliness and to help bridge the gap that exists between older adults and technology use. Not only do these calls provide social stimulation, but wellness callers are also able to connect participants to a variety of community resources. SBP has helped connect individuals to COVID-19 related information, food assistance, transportation, and provided various forms of technological support.

Between March 2020 and February 2022, the team has made 1304 wellness check-in calls. Of those calls, 658 led to what were considered productive conversations, and 78 percent of these left participants reporting that they felt 'significantly better' due to receiving the call. Some interactions led to outcomes that greatly affected the lives of our participants. One participant who was houseless was assisted in developing a social media platform for their business. Another participant took advantage of SBP assistance to shift their therapy practice to telehealth, allowing them to continue working through the pandemic. These are just two examples of positive outcomes stemming from SBP support.

In the summer of 2021, a survey was conducted in order to gather data from SBP participants about their experience in the program [58]. Participants were offered the chance to provide feedback and reflect with the survey provider. A number of quotes are listed below highlighting the significant impact the Social Bridging Project had on some of its participants.

"The other day I was having a really, *really* bad day. I've got psychiatric issues. It was one of those days where my mental health providers were not giving me what I needed. I really needed someone to talk to help me get grounded. I didn't tell [caller] I was having a crisis because I knew he would tell me to call my therapist, but he helped me a lot."

"It made me feel like [loneliness] was a recognized problem. It wasn't just my problem. Back in my grandmother's time she had family around her, and it was a community where she could walk from one family to the next."

"It made me feel like I could have a part of the future; that she and also the program thought that geriatric people were important enough to have this program."

"The non-threatening way to get my tech questions answered. And it's very expensive to hire somebody to help with tech. Without your program I never would have made it this far.... Your program is worth its weight in gold. It has been invaluable in getting me to think outside the box."

These quotes illustrate the ways in which the Social Bridging Project participants were being affected by the program. Not only were practical solutions found for the needs of the participants, but positive emotional outcomes and feelings of social support were also experienced. One participant even notes the improved outlook they had on society as an older adult after feeling included by SBP.

4.3 Recommendation 3: medical providers and health teams should build on efforts to reach people in their homes or communities with whole person medical and health care

In-home medical care is infamous for being difficult to access due to issues with availability or cost. Policies aimed at bolstering payments for in-home and community-based caregiving, such as that proposed as part of President Biden's "Build Back Better" infrastructure bill, would provide a much-needed pathway to improving older Americans' access to these services that are often essential to aging in place. Infusing more dollars into programs that support the direct care workforce for older adults living at home is also likely to improve the quality and availability of care provided.

Furthermore, efforts should be made to improve the financial feasibility of programs shown to benefit multiple dimensions of older adult wellbeing, such as home-based primary care, through advocacy for value-based payment models or risk-sharing arrangements. As it currently stands, Medicare's standard fee-for-service structure has not adopted value-based reimbursement principles, and this has a significant impact on the ability of medical practices to offer this impactful service in a way that is financially sustainable.

Finally, enhanced reimbursement for telemedicine visits, particularly phone visits, would allow clinicians to continue providing medical care, behavioral health support, medication management, etc. for older adults with barriers to either in-office visits (e.g., due to transportation difficulties) or video telehealth visits (e.g., due to broadband or technology access) while maintaining clinical solvency. In their chapter on telemedicine and telehealth, Chiang, and co-authors state "Advances in telecommunication technologies have introduced many ways to bridge geographic distance and time, in order to connect clinicians, patients and families and facilitate the remote delivery of health care services and education" [59]. This is important to ensure that socially isolated older patients, already at increased risk of adverse health events by virtue of their isolation, do not also suffer substantial gaps in medical care for their chronic health conditions that would further exacerbate their risk.

4.4 Recommendation 4: broad public (community and governmental) support for infrastructure and technology access and education projects is needed

Large, publicly funded infrastructure projects are needed to expand broadband access in rural areas. Technology and education projects will help to bridge the digital divide and bring medical and social support to people in rural areas and to those unable to leave their homes safely or easily. Policies and projects that bridge the digital divide especially for rural places and older adults or others socially isolated in their living situations are important. While interventions to increase digital access may not satisfactorily replace in-person interaction, they can help to supplement communication during times when face-to-face connection with other individuals is not possible.

Emergency policies put in place during the early months of the pandemic increased the ability of health care providers to deliver and bill for a wide variety of virtual visits (telehealth) including medical, psychiatric, specialist, dental, orthopedic, pharmacy and other services [60, 61]. While there are some disadvantages to the more widespread use of telemedicine that was brought on by the pandemic, many believe the benefits outweigh the drawbacks [62]. Key advantages of telemedicine include its cost effectiveness, the extension of access to specialty services, and the possibility of reducing the impact of a looming shortage of doctors especially in rural settings. In order to realize the promise of telemedicine and be prepared for future public health emergencies, policy makers need to expand technological resources into rural places, and health care providers need "to fully immerse telemedicine services into the healthcare landscape" [62].

For people who have not grown up with computers, smartphones, and other handheld digital technologies, increasing access to telecommunication capabilities needs to be paired with opportunities to learn how to use these technologies. A case example of a technology education and support program from western NC is the App State Cyber-Seniors program. In collaboration with the international Cyber-Seniors© organization, the program pairs Appalachian State University students with local older adults to teach digital and technology literacy skills such as the use of devices or video conference platforms, and to find resources for online education and local, remotely delivered resources and support. The program is designed to support social reciprocity (between students and elders) and to close the digital divide while reducing social isolation and loneliness among adults living in a mountainous rural region of the state [63].

4.5 Recommendation 5: public health efforts should center place and use a place-based approach to addressing social isolation and other health and social determinants of health concerns

Although social isolation and its health impacts are global phenomena, and some strategies such as provision of technology infrastructure and support for policies that prioritize social connectedness will have broad applicability, the efforts to address social connectedness as a social determinant of health should be specific to place. A place-based approach means taking the context of place, community and people's experience including history, culture, norms, and stories into account as policies, programs, and actions are planned. According to a WNC-located Master of Public Health Program in Asheville, "[p]lace-based public health centers people and their communities as the catalyst for transforming systems to promote wellbeing for all. Local residents, not institutions, hold the history, knowledge, and ways of interacting with place. As such, a place's inhabitants and institutions work in relationship, using interdisciplinary and participatory processes, to create and lead efforts to sustainably improve the social drivers of health and ultimately actualize health equity."

By utilizing a place-based approach, public health teams are more likely to address community and public health in ways that enact health equity in systems, organizations, and communities.

An excellent example of how centering place in public health efforts can be seen in community health worker (CHW) networks. Community health workers (CHWs) are increasingly important players in supporting the health of people where they live, worship, work, eat and play. CHWs are trained lay persons who generally come from and reside in the community where they work, who provide culturally relevant health information, help people access the resources and care they need, provide informal guidance, and advocate for community health needs among other activities [64]. CHWs often connect with people in their homes or in community settings, adding to social connection while supporting access to health care or social determinant of health needs, and this approach could be a valuable way to support older adults experiencing loneliness, social isolation and many other mental, physical, or technological needs.

In 2021, the NC Center for Health and Wellness in partnership with Mountain Area Health Education Center and community-based organizations conducted a mixed methods evaluation of the "Community Health Workers as Culturally-Responsive COVID Support in WNC Communities" initiative to explore the impact and quality of CHW services across 17 counties over the yearlong period. Across the methods used, the research team saw significant impacts of the community health workers, particularly in rural communities and among "hidden" or "abandoned" and hard-to-serve groups. While the research did not focus on older adults, several of the findings related to the CHW's impacts on health and social determinants highlight the importance of a place-based approach and could be particularly important among isolated older adults.

CHWs participated in a focus group and responded to a survey to share the services they provided and their perceptions of their impact. One CHW described the incredible range of services she provided (30 in total), which were for both health issues and social determinants and meeting urgent needs. One CHW shared that she felt the social connections she made were particularly important: "It is a pleasure to be able to help these people and to see the smiles on their faces and to see what they achieve...you have a connection with these people that you see every day" (2021 CHW Focus Group). Another said making connections in the community and building trust was incredibly important: "they open their door, and they open their lives to us" (2021 CHW Focus Group).

Community-based researchers also interviewed community members who had received CHW services, and the list of services and resources they reported receiving from CHWs was extensive. Services included COVID-related resources such as educational information, personal protective equipment (PPE), hand sanitizer, cleaning supplies, and vaccine information. While many community members found these resources and supplies important, most also received non COVID-related help, which they really valued. These resources included connection to housing, transportation, connection with Pisgah Legal for health insurance assistance, referrals to financial programs, connection with food stamps, food boxes, rental assistance, medication assistance, and help paying bills. Housing and transportation were resources that were most mentioned by community members, with housing lifted up as being a resource that there just is not enough of in Western North Carolina. An additional resource that many community members reported receiving was emotional support. This emotional support felt especially important to many, as they may or may not have had others in their lives to provide this: "it's good to have somebody, especially if you don't have nobody to come around" (September 2021 Interview). CHWs were often described as becoming members of the family. These connections were valuable to community members because they generally made them feel better and sometimes helped them to feel less isolated and alone.

Continued and expanded investment in Community Health Workers as vital members of the healthcare workforce could help meet community members' health, emotional and social needs.

5. Conclusions

Social isolation is an important concern among older adults and is associated with poor health outcomes. Older adults have been disproportionately impacted by increases in social isolation exacerbated by COVID-19 pandemic mitigation policies and efforts. For these reasons three broad-based recommendations should be employed at the at the county, state, and country levels. Social isolation and its antidote, social connectedness, should be recognized as a social determinant of health. Governments at all levels should legislate and support for broad band access and technology infrastructure. And, public health efforts should center place and use a place-based approach to addressing social isolation, healthy equity, and other health and social determinants of health concerns. In addition, more localized support is necessary to turn the tide on the widespread impact of social isolation on the health of older adults. State, county, and local policy makers, human service organizations, and funders must prioritize programmatic opportunities to increase social connection for older adults. These efforts will need to include education and ongoing support for the use of digital technologies. Finally, medical providers and health teams should build on efforts to reach people in their homes or communities with whole person medical and health care. Projects and practices in western NC may serve as a model for implementation of these recommendations in other places.

Acknowledgements

This work was supported by a grant from the Dogwood Health Trust. The authors wish to acknowledge the following individuals for their contributions, Ellen Bailey, Nadia Mazza, Jill Juris Naar, and Katie Cox.

Conflict of interest

The authors declare no conflicts of interest.

Author details

Amy Joy Lanou[1*], Jeff Jones[2], Louise Noble[2], Thomas Smythe[2], Lauren Alexa Gambrill[3], Emma Olson[2] and Tasha Woodall[4,5]

1 NC Center for Health and Wellness and UNC Asheville – UNC Gillings Master of Public Health Program, University of North Carolina Asheville, Asheville, North Carolina, USA

2 NC Center for Health and Wellness, University of North Carolina Asheville, Asheville, North Carolina, USA

3 University of Washington, Seattle, Washington, USA

4 Mountain Area Health Education Center, Asheville, North Carolina, USA

5 UNC Eshelman School of Pharmacy, UNC School of Medicine, Chapel Hill, NC, USA

*Address all correspondence to: alanou@unca.edu

References

[1] Medicine NA of S Engineering, and, Education D of B and SS and, Division H and M, Sciences B on B Cognitive, and Sensory, Policy B on HS, Adults C on the H and MD of SI and L in O. Social Isolation and Loneliness in Older Adults: Opportunities for the Health Care System. Washington, DC: National Academies Press; 2020

[2] Holt-Lunstad J, Smith TB, Layton JB. Social relationships and mortality risk: A Meta-analytic review. PLoS Medicine. 2010;**7**(7):e1000316. DOI: 10.1371/journal.pmed.1000316

[3] Fakoya OA, McCorry NK, Donnelly M. Loneliness and social isolation interventions for older adults: A scoping review of reviews. BMC Public Health. 2020,**20**.1. DOI: 10.1186/s12889-020-8251-6

[4] Latikka R, Rubio-Hernández R, Lohan ES, Rantala J, Fernández FN, Laitinen A, et al. Older adults' loneliness, social isolation, and physical information and communication technology in the era of ambient assisted living: A systematic literature review. Journal of Medical Internet Research. 2021;**23**(12):e28022. DOI: 10.2196/28022

[5] Gao Q, Prina AM, Prince M, Acosta D, Sosa AL, Guerra M, et al. Loneliness among older adults in latin america, China, and India: Prevalence, correlates and association with mortality. International Journal of Public Health. 2021;**66**:604449. DOI: 10.3389/ijph.2021.604449

[6] National Academies of Sciences, Engineering, and Medicine. Social Isolation and Loneliness in Older Adults: Opportunities for the Health Care System. Washington, DC: The National Academies Press; 2020. DOI: 10.17226/25663

[7] Australian Government. Australian Institute of Health and Welfare. Ageing and Aged Care [Internet]. 2017. Available from: https://www.aihw.gov.au/getmedia/d18a1d2b-692c-42bf-81e2-47cd54c51e8d/aihw-australias-welfare-2017-chapter5-1.pdf.aspx#:~:text=It%20is%20estimated%20that%20around,2016

[8] EU Science Hub. How Lonely Are Europeans? The European Commission's Science and Knowledge Service [Internet]. 2019, June. Available from: https://ec.europa.eu/jrc/en/news/how-lonely-are-europeans

[9] Stickley A, Koyanagi A. Physical multimorbidity and loneliness: A population-based study. PLoS One. 2018;**13**(1):e0191651-e0191651. DOI: 10.1371/journal.pone.0191651

[10] Hawkley LC, Cacioppo JT. Loneliness matters: A theoretical and empirical review of consequences and mechanisms. Annals of Behavioral Medicine. 2010;**40**(2):218-227. DOI: 10.1007/s12160-010-9210-8

[11] Holt-Lunstad J, Smith TB, Baker M, Harris T, Stephenson D. Loneliness and social isolation as risk factors for mortality: A meta-analytic review. Perspectives on Psychological Science. 2015;**10**(2):227-237. DOI: 10.1177/1745691614568352

[12] Anderson M, Perrin, A. Tech adoption climbs among older adults [Internet]. 2017. Pew Research Center. Available from: https://www.pewresearch.org/internet/wp-content/uploads/sites/9/2017/05/PI_2017.05.17_Older-Americans-Tech_FINAL.pdf

[13] Graham J. Technology Divide Between Senior "Haves" and

"Have-Nots" Roils Pandemic Response [Internet]. 2020. KHN. Available from: https://khn.org/news/technology-divide-between-senior-haves-and-have-nots-roils-pandemic-response/

[14] Shteinlukht T. COVID-19 Pandemia impact on mental health of older adults and possible treatment options. The American Journal of Geriatric Psychiatry. 2021;**29**(4):S102-S103

[15] Perrin A. Digital gap between rural and nonrural America persists [Internet]. 2019. Pew Research Center. Available from: https://www.pewresearch.org/fact-tank/2019/05/31/digital-gap-between-rural-andnonrural-america-persists/

[16] US Census Bureau. Data census [Internet]. 2021

[17] North Carolina Office of State Budget and Management. The Urban and Rural Faces of North Carolina [Internet]. 2021, July. North Carolina Government. Available from: https://files.nc.gov/ncosbm/documents/files/2018ACSNC.pdf

[18] Henning-Smith C, Moscovice I, Kozhimannil K. Differences in social isolation and its relationship to health by rurality. The Journal of Rural Health. 2019;**35**(4):540-549. DOI: 10.1111/jrh.12344

[19] Henning-Smith C. Meeting the social needs of older adults in rural areas. JAMA Health Forum. 2020;**1**(11):e201411. DOI: 10.1001/jamahealthforum.2020.1411

[20] Kaur H . Why rural Americans are having a hard time working from home [Internet]. 2020, April 29. CNN. Available from: https://www.cnn.com/2020/04/29/us/rural-broadband-accesscoronavirus-trnd/index.html

[21] Hamilton J. Maybe isolation, not loneliness, shortens life. Shots: Health news from NPR [Internet]. Available from: http://www.npr.org/sections/health-shots/2013/03/26/175283008/maybe-isolation-not-loneliness-shortens-life [Accessed July 22, 2015]

[22] Henning-Smith C. The unique impact of COVID-19 on older adults in rural areas. Journal of Aging & Social Policy. 2020;**32**(4-5):396-402

[23] World Health Organization. Social determinants of health. Available from: https://www.who.int/westernpacific/health-topics/social-determinants-of-health

[24] Santoli JM. Effects of the COVID-19 pandemic on routine Pediatric vaccine ordering and administration — United States. MMWR. Morbidity and Mortality Weekly Report. 2020;**69**:591-593. DOI: 10.15585/mmwr.mm6919e2

[25] Moreland A. Timing of state and territorial COVID-19 stay-at-home orders and changes in population movement — United States. MMWR. Morbidity and Mortality Weekly Report. 2020;**69**:1198-1203. DOI: 10.15585/mmwr.mm6935a2

[26] Fisher KA. Factors associated with cloth face covering use among adults during the COVID-19 pandemic — United States. MMWR. Morbidity and Mortality Weekly Report. 2020;**69**:933-937. DOI: 10.15585/mmwr.mm6928e3

[27] Wright AL, Chawla G, Chen L, Farmer A. Tracking mask mandates during the Covid-19 pandemic. Social Science Research Network. 2020:1-14. DOI: 10.2139/ssrn.3667149

[28] Chu DK, Akl EA, Duda S, et al. Physical distancing, face masks, and eye protection to prevent person-to-person transmission of SARS-CoV-2 and COVID-19: A systematic review and meta-analysis.

Lancet. 2020;**395**(10242):1973-1987. DOI: 10.1016/S0140-6736(20)31142-9

[29] Badr HS, Du H, Marshall M, Dong E, Squire MM, Gardner LM. Association between mobility patterns and COVID-19 transmission in the USA: A mathematical modelling study. The Lancet Infectious Diseases. 2020;**20**(11):1247-1254. DOI: 10.1016/S1473-3099(20)30553-

[30] Galea S, Merchant RM, Lurie N. The mental health consequences of COVID-19 and physical distancing: The need for prevention and early intervention. JAMA Internal Medicine. 2020;**180**(6):817-818. DOI: 10.1001/jamainternmed.2020.1562

[31] CDC. Cases, Data, and Surveillance. Centers for Disease Control and Prevention [Internet]. February 11, 2020. Available from: https://www.cdc.gov/coronavirus/2019-ncov/covid-data/investigations-discovery/hospitalization-death-by-age.html

[32] Bruine de Bruin W. Age differences in COVID-19 Risk perceptions and mental health: Evidence from a National U.S. survey conducted in March 2020. The Journals of Gerontology: Series B. Feb 2021;**76**(2):e24-e29. DOI: 10.1093/geronb/gbaa074

[33] Hadjistavropoulos T, Asmundson GJG. COVID stress in older adults: Considerations during the omicron wave and beyond. Journal of Anxiety Disorders. 2022;**86**:102535. DOI: 10.1016/j.janxdis.2022.102535

[34] Santini ZI, Jose PE, York Cornwell E, et al. Social disconnectedness, perceived isolation, and symptoms of depression and anxiety among older Americans (NSHAP): A longitudinal mediation analysis. The Lancet Public Health. 2020;**5**(1):e62-e70. DOI: 10.1016/S2468-2667(19)30230-0

[35] Roe CM, Rosnick CB, Colletta A, Babulal GM. Reaction to a pandemic: Social distancing and driving among older adults during COVID-19. Journal of Applied Gerontology. 2021;**40**(3):263-267. DOI: 10.1177/0733464820966516

[36] Flint AJ, Bingham KS, Iaboni A. Effect of COVID-19 on the mental health care of older people in Canada. International Psychogeriatrics. 2020;**32**(10):1113-1116. DOI: 10.1017/S1041610220000708

[37] Nicholson NR. A review of social isolation: An important but underassessed condition in older adults. The Journal of Primary Prevention. 2012;**33**(2-3):137-152 Available from: https://link.springer.com/content/pdf/10.1007/s10935-012-0271-2.pdf

[38] Freedman VA, Hu M, Kasper JD. Changes in older adults' social contact during the COVID-19 pandemic. Journals of Gerontology - Series B Psychological Sciences and Social Sciences. 2021 Sep 16:gbab166. DOI: 10.1093/geronb/gbab166. Epub ahead of print

[39] Cortez C, Mansour O, Qato DM, Stafford RS, Alexander GC. Changes in short-term, long-term, and preventive care delivery in US Office-based and telemedicine visits during the COVID-19 pandemic. JAMA Health Forum. 2021;**2**(7):e211529. DOI: 10.1001/jamahealthforum.2021.1529

[40] Eberly LA, Kallan MJ, Julien HM, et al. Patient characteristics associated with telemedicine access for primary and specialty ambulatory care during the COVID-19 pandemic. JAMA Network Open. 2020;**3**(12):e2031640. DOI: 10.1001/jamanetworkopen.2020.31640

[41] Hunsaker A, Hargittai E. A review of internet use among older adults. New

Media & Society. 2018;**20**(10):3937-3954. DOI: 10.1177/1461444818787348

[42] Wang JY, Bennett K, Probst J. Subdividing the digital divide: Differences in internet access and use among rural residents with medical limitations. Journal of Medical Internet Research. 2011;**13**(1):e1534. DOI: 10.2196/jmir.1534

[43] Woodall T, Ramage M, LaBruyere JT, McLean W, Tak CR. Telemedicine services during COVID-19: Considerations for medically underserved populations. The Journal of Rural Health. 2021;**37**(1):231-234

[44] Chodosh J, Weinstein BE, Blustein J. Face masks can be devastating for people with hearing loss. BMJ. 2020;**370**:m2683. DOI: 10.1136/bmj.m2683

[45] Nguyen DD, McCabe P, Thomas D, et al. Acoustic voice characteristics with and without wearing a facemask. Scientific Reports. 2021;**11**(1):5651. DOI: 10.1038/s41598-021-85130-8

[46] Brown B. The Gifts of Imperfection: Let Go of Who you Think you're Supposed to be and Embrace Who you Are. Center City, Minnesota: Hazeldon; 2010

[47] Baumeister RF, Leary MR. The need to belong: Desire for interpersonal attachments as a fundamental human motivation. Psychological Bulletin. 1995;**117**(3):497-529. DOI: 10.1037/0033-2909.117.3.497

[48] Burleson MH, Roberts NA, Munson AA, Duncan CJ, Randall AK, Ha T, et al. Feeling the absence of touch: Distancing, distress, regulation, and relationships in the context of COVID-19. Journal of Social and Personal Relationships. 2022;**39**(1):56-79. DOI: 10.1177/02654075211052696

[49] Lindsay Smith G, Banting L, Eime R, O'Sullivan G, van Uffelen JGZ. The association between social support and physical activity in older adults: A systematic review. International Journal of Behavioral Nutrition and Physical Activity. 2017;**14**:56. DOI: 10.1186/s12966-017-0509-8

[50] Berkman LF, Kawachi I, Glymour MM. Social capital, social cohesion, and health. In: Social Epidemiology. Oxford, England: Oxford University Press; 2014

[51] Cotman CW, Berchtold NC, Christie LA. Exercise builds brain health: Key roles of growth factor cascades and inflammation. Trends in Neurosciences. 2007;**30**(9):464-472. DOI: 10.1016/j.tins.2007.06.011. Epub 2007 Aug 31. Erratum in: Trends Neurosci. 2007 Oct;30(10):489. PMID: 17765329

[52] De Felicis J. 13 Unusual Ways to Shed Stress (Lessons from the World's Blue Zones) - Blue Zones [Internet]. 2022. Available from: https://www.bluezones.com/2022/02/13-unusual-ways-to-shed-stress-lessons-from-the-worlds-blue-zones/

[53] Emlet CA, Moceri JT. The importance of social connectedness in building age-friendly communities. Journal of Aging Research. 2012;**2012**:173247. DOI: 10.1155/2012/173247

[54] Lee NT. Public Policy Can Improve Older Adults' Access to Technology. Washington, DC: The Brookings Institution; 2017. Available from: https://www.brookings.edu/blog/techtank/2017/06/05/public-policy-can-improve-older-adults-access-to-technology/

[55] Fang Y, Chau AKC, Wong A, Fung HH, Woo J. Information and communicative technology use enhances psychological well-being of older adults: The roles

of age, social connectedness, and frailty status. Aging & Mental Health. 2018;**22**(11):1516-1524. DOI: 10.1080/13607863.2017.1358354

[56] Cotten SR. Examining the roles of Technology in Aging and Quality of life. The Journals of Gerontology. Series B, Psychological Sciences and Social Sciences. 2017;**72**(5):823-826. DOI: 10.1093/geronb/gbx109

[57] Suragarn U, Hain D, Pfaff G. Approaches to enhance social connection in older adults: An integrative review of literature. Aging and Health Research. 2021;**1**(3):100029. DOI: 10.1016/j.ahr.2021.100029

[58] Noble LW, Olson E, Woodall T, Jones J, Smythe T, Whitlock C, et al. The social bridging project: Intergenerational phone-based connections with older adults during the COVID-19 pandemic. Gerontology and Geriatric Medicine. 2022 Apr 4;**8**:23337214221083473. 1-10. DOI: 10.1177/23337214221083473

[59] Chiang MF, Starren JB, Demiris G. In: Shortliffe EH, Cimino JJ, editors. Telemedicine and Telehealth. Cham: Biomedical Informatics. Springer; 2021. DOI: 10.1007/978-3-030-58721-5_20

[60] Public Health Institute Center for Connected Health Policy. State Telehealth Laws & Reimbursement Policies [Internet]. 2020. Available from: https://www.cchpca.org/sites/default/files/2020-05/CCHP_%2050_STATE_REPORT_SPRING_2020_FINAL.pdf

[61] Turner Lee N, Karsten J, Roberts J. Removing regulatory barriers to telehealth before and after COVID-19 [Internet]. 2020..Brookings Institution. Available from: https://www.brookings.edu/research/removing-regulatory-barriers-to-telehealth-before-and-after-covid-19

[62] Kichloo A, Albosta M, Dettloff K, et al. Telemedicine, the current COVID-19 pandemic and the future: A narrative review and perspectives moving forward in the USA. Family Medicine and Community Health. 2020;**8**:e000530. DOI: 10.1136/fmch-2020-000530

[63] Appalachian State AppState Cyber-Seniors [Internet]. 2021. Available from: https://ihhs.appstate.edu/outreach/appstate-cyber-seniors

[64] U.S. Department of Health and Human Services, Health Resources and Services Administration, Bureau of Health Professions. (2007). Community Health Worker National Workforce Study. Washington, DC: US Department of Health and Human Services; 2007

Section 3

Novel Approaches to Prevention and Treatment of Age-Related Declines

Chapter 6

Perspective Chapter: The Role of Modifiable Factors, Particularly Nutritional Factors, on Age-Related Sarcopenia

Nafiseh Shokri-Mashhadi

Abstract

Advances in medicine result in an increase in the age of global population. The percentage of people over 60 years will approximately be duplicated up to 22 between 2015 and 2050, which is associated with a notable rise in age-related complications such as sarcopenia and frailty. The age-related sarcopenia is defined by low muscle strength, and it is considered severe if low muscle strength, low muscle mass, and low physical performance are detected.This condition is associated with poor quality of life, risk of falls, fractures, and higher healthcare costs. Despite the growing interest regarding the treatment of this phenomenon, the lack of adequate knowledge underlying the multifactorial parthenogenesis of age-related sarcopenia hinders the diagnosis of effective therapeutic approaches. In this respect, one of the major solutions would be to recognize the effect of modifiable factors on muscle health during the lifetime. Previous observations indicated that dietary and nutritional factors, beyond other environmental agents across the life course are related to muscle mass and function in the elderly. With respect to the fundamental role of nutrients with antioxidants properties in maintaining many aspects of health, this chapter aims to discuss the association between components of sarcopenia and nutritional status in older adults, and their potential effect on prevention and treatment of age-related sarcopenia.

Keywords: age-related sarcopenia, nutritional factors, prevention, treatment, dietary quality

1. Introduction

1.1 Definition of sarcopenia

The average age of populations is increasing because of numerous factors, including advances in medical care and decreasing birth rate [1, 2]. The percentage of people over 60 years will approximately be duplicated up to 22 between 2015 and 2050, which is associated with a notable rise in age-related complications such as sarcopenia and frailty [3]. Definitions of age-related sarcopenia have evolved over time in an attempt to better characterize sarcopenia. The name for this phenomenon derives from the Greek term sarx (flesh) and penia (loss) [4]. Early definitions of sarcopenia were based exclusively on an age-related reduction in muscle mass [5]. However, the two-dimensional nature of these conditions (muscle mass loss and muscle strength loss) suggests that both its quantitative and qualitative range should be evaluated [6]. Therefore, the European Working Group on Sarcopenia in Older People (EWGSOP) described sarcopenia as an age-associated decline in muscle mass and strength with functional impairment [7].

Beyond the loss of muscle tissue that occurs over a lifetime, this condition is also associated with the conversion of type II fibers to type I fibers, which results in impairment of muscle quality and muscle function [8].

Categorizing sarcopenia into pre-sarcopenia, sarcopenia, and severe sarcopenia has also been defined by the EWGSOP that suggested the pre-sarcopenia stage as low muscle mass with no impact on muscle strength or physical performance, whereas the sarcopenia stage distinguished as low muscle mass with either low muscle strength or low physical performance and severe sarcopenia as the presence of all three criteria [9]. While interest in sarcopenia has risen in recent years, contention still exists over most components of the disease, with a universally accepted definition still lacking.

1.2 Diagnosis of sarcopenia

Various approaches can be used to assess muscle mass. Current assessment tools include body imaging techniques, bioelectric impedance analysis, anthropometric parameters, and biochemical markers [10].

Computed tomography (CT) and magnetic resonance imaging are able to effectively distinguish fat from other soft tissues, which makes these presently the gold standard method for the assessment of body composition. However, limited access, the high cost, and the risk of radiation inhibit the use of these techniques in clinical practice [11]. Therefore, dual-energy X-ray absorptiometry (DXA) is the most popular method for correctly evaluating body composition and widely used to assess muscle mass in research studies due to speed of measurement and relatively low per patient scan cost with typically low radiation [12]. Though, seeking for inexpensive, easy-to-use, and derived measures methods such as phase angle causes the application of bioimpedance technology. Nevertheless, using the estimation of body composition and muscle mass through anthropometric measurements, such as mid-upper arm circumference, calf circumference, and skinfold thickness, may allow us initially assess sarcopenia in situations that imaging equipment is typically unavailable in primary care settings [13].

The defining cutoff point for the identification of muscle loss depends upon the measurement technique chosen and the availability of reference studies. Low muscle mass is usually distinguished by a skeletal muscle mass index ranging from 7.23 kg/m2 to 8.87 kg/m2 in men and 5.45 kg/m2 to 6.42 kg/m2 in women [14]. Moreover, it is generally accepted that low physical performance is defined as a gait speed of less than 0.8 m/sec [15] and low muscle strength is usually defined by handgrip strength of less than 30 kg for men and less than 20 kg for women [7]. Nevertheless, the quadriceps strength cut-off points of 18.0 kg for older men and 16.0 kg for older women proposed as a muscle strength measurement for sarcopenia diagnosis in older Asian people [16].

Because of this diversity in the cutoffs of the sarcopenia's characterization, EWGSOP has recommended that more research is urgently needed in order to obtain accurate reference values for different nations and countries around the world [17].

1.3 Pathophysiology of and risk factors for sarcopenia

The pathophysiology of sarcopenia is multifactorial. Several underlying mechanisms have been linked to the development of sarcopenia, although not all have been fully elucidated [6]. Prevalence of sarcopenia is mostly associated with chronic inflammation, which may lead to a vicious cycle of intricate interactions among risk factors [18]. However, research on sarcopenia prevention and treatment is developing quickly because of insufficient evidence for the underlying cellular mechanisms of the progress and maintenance of sarcopenia. So, it seems that understanding the factors related to increasing sarcopenia risk may provide strategies for intervention and disease improvement.

Inflammation in aging is one of the main suggested factors of sarcopenia characterized by a chronic progressive increase in pro-inflammatory cytokines, and the reduced serum level of anti-inflammatory cytokines [17]. Decline in immune function, plays an important role in several age-related diseases, for example Alzheimer's disease, Parkinson's disease, multiple sclerosis, atherosclerosis, and other complications [19, 20].

The majority of studies have demonstrated that inflammatory cytokines have an important effect on skeletal muscle wasting, leading to an imbalance between protein synthesis and catabolism [21]. It reasonably has shown that reduced rates of protein synthesis paralleled to increased protein breakdown in the skeletal muscle are associated with a variety of produced pro-inflammatory cytokines during the inflammatory response. Indeed, the effects of pro-inflammatory cytokines on muscle mass may be mediated by activating the transcription factor NF-κB in line with a production of ROS in the muscle of the elderly people [22, 23]. Additionally, we recently indicated that circulating levels of C-reactive protein (CRP) and hs-CRP are independently associated with impairment of muscle strength [24]. It is also suggested that low muscle strength is associated with the high levels of inflammatory cytokines [25] such as CRP [26]. These findings may suggest that the plasma concentration of some inflammatory molecules is related to the aspects of muscle decline and functional impairment.

Another suggested factor is Insulin resistance (IR) which is defined by reduced peripheral glucose utilization in skeletal muscle, majority of whole-body insulin-stimulated glucose disposal, that develops with age [27]. Various studies demonstrated that IR is related markedly to the different diagnostic components of sarcopenia [28]. Data on the prevalence of sarcopenia in Korean elderly men aged more than 65 years recommended that higher IR and lower vitamin D levels are independently associated with the presence of sarcopenia in community-dwelling elderly men [29]. In another study conducted by Gorshunova et al., low muscle mass and muscle strength were significantly related to increased indices of IR, probably as a result of energy homeostasis disorders and the deterioration of glucose in the skeletal muscles [30]. One of the anticipated mechanisms of insulin resistance in elderly people is a reduction in the size of type II fibers which may reduce mitochondrial activity and result in IR in muscle [31, 32].

On the other hand, recent investigations illustrated that serum level of negative regulator of muscle growth, such as myostatin could increase with advancing age [33] and may play an important role in the resistance of insulin in muscles [34]. Moreover, aging skeletal muscle inflammation through activation of the classical signaling pathway also has impact on insulin uptake [35]. Furthermore, the effect of accumulation of intramyocellular lipid has been systematically evaluated and reported a well-established association between accumulation of intramyocellular lipid and muscle IR [30]. Finally, it is understood that strategies for identifying improvements and insulin sensitivity treatments can propose possible preventive measures against sarcopenia.

Aging is also related to changes in a several hormones status, including testosterone, estrogen, growth hormone, insulin-like growth factor 1, and corticosteroids [36], and the clinical significance of these deficiencies is variable with age [37]. It is previously supposed that the age-dependent decline in GH and IGF-1 levels is related to the pathogenesis of sarcopenia [38]. Moreover, in a recent observational cohort study, low baseline serum IGF-1 levels correlated with lower handgrip strength and worse physical performance [39]. Nevertheless, the impact of long-term GH therapy in the treatment of sarcopenia in elderly individuals with low GH/IGF-1 levels is still unclear. Cortisol is also the most potent immunosuppressive agent which can be stimulated by inflammation and therefore can be related to the development of sarcopenia and its components; muscle strength, muscle mass, and physical function. We could speculate from studies that the systemic overproduction of glucocorticoids during aging is associated with an increase of sarcopenia risk. However, further longitudinal studies are required to confirm these relationships.

In terms of modifiable risk factors, the relationship between adult lifestyle and sarcopenia has been highlighted in order to provide strategies for prevention of and improvement in age-related sarcopenia. In this concern, mental state, smoking, low body mass index (BMI), nutritional status, and physical activities have been introduced as the most potential changeable factors that could be applied in future strategies to prevent or delay the progression of sarcopenia [40–42]. The strong association between alteration in body composition in lifetime, namely fat-free mass, skeletal muscle mass, and BMI with prevalence and incidence of sarcopenia has been shown [43]. In addition, various previous reviews of studies revealed the relationship between physical inactivity and losses of muscle mass and strength [40], while resistance training was reported to have a beneficial effect on the physical performance measures in most studies [44, 45]. Regarding mental health, several studies found that sarcopenia is associated with cognitive decline and depression which could be due to some of the predisposing factors underlying sarcopenia, such as oxidative stress, inflammation, and insulin resistance [46]. Among them, one of the important modifiable factors in maintaining healthy status, in helping recovery from acute conditions, and in prevention of chronic diseases across lifespan is optimal nutritional status [47]. On the other hand, poor nutritional status is associated with several adverse consequences in community-dwelling older individuals, such as inflammation, cachexia, altered gut integrity, and muscle dysfunction [48, 49]. In addition, it is shown that the quality of the diet along with the lifetime has a close relationship with the sarcopenia [50]. It has been demonstrated that individuals consuming less energy will lose more muscle tissue. Therefore, avoiding under-nutrition is required to prevent muscle loss [47, 51]. Many nutrients have also been linked with the development of sarcopenia [47]. In this regard, the Korea National Health and Nutrition Examination Survey (KNHANES) cohort has revealed a lower energy, protein, and carbohydrate intake among sarcopenic older adults [52]. Given that evaluating the role of dietary nutrient intake in the treatment and development of sarcopenia would be valuable. Following we summarized studies in which the role of various nutritional factors on age-related sarcopenia was evaluated.

2. Role of nutritional factors in prevention and treatment of sarcopenia

2.1 Role of dietary protein in prevention and treatment of sarcopenia

The scientific literature indicated that the amount of daily protein intake is related to prevention of muscle functional decline and sarcopenia treatment, as older adults have an increased need for dietary protein to stimulate their muscle protein synthesis [53, 54]. Furthermore, Sovianne et al., showed a significant difference in protein intake (gram/day) among sarcopenic and non-sarcopenic older adults [55]. It is supposed that lower energy requirements and reduced appetite decrease total energy consumption in aging, which can significantly reduce dietary intake of protein [56]. It proposed that dietary protein supplementation more than recommended dietary intake (above 0.8 g/kg/d) may have beneficial effect on sarcopenia [57, 58]. However, other recent studies have shown that muscle loss cannot be entirely stopped, even when daily protein intake is maintained at a high level [59]. So, the role of protein supplementation on age-related sarcopenia is somewhat controversial and might be affected by the nutritional status of individuals [60].

It is also worth noting that the type of protein ingested and timing of protein intake throughout the day could determine the amount of skeletal muscle mass [61]. In these regards,nutritional supplementation including 20 g whey protein and 800 IU vitamin D in previous randomized double blind research leads to further losses of intermuscular fat ($p = .049$) and increased normal muscle density ($p = .018$) after the 6-month intervention [62]. These results were also confirmed by another study [63]. However, a recent meta-analysis of eight studies (n = 557) conducted by Tieland et al., showed no significant positive effects of protein or amino acid supplementation on lean body mass, muscle strength, or handgrip. Nevertheless, it seems that there were various heterogeneities in included trials in the mentioned study, such as duration of treatment and type of supplementation, and dosage which could affect the result interpretation [64]. So, it can be concluded that this general lack of effect of protein supplements directed us to assess positive associations between protein intake and muscle mass and function through cohort studies.

The anabolic effects of some amino acids on muscle mass also have been investigated in several studies. Creatine, as one of the most important amino acids located primarily in muscle tissue, accelerates muscle ATP regeneration throughout the increased energy demand [65, 66]. In this aera, the increased muscle mass and muscle strength with exercises and an additional effect of creatine were found in clinical trials [67]. Moreover, increased physical performance with exercises and an interactive effect of creatine were observed in some studies [68]. Results of a previous meta-analyses specified that creatine supplementation combined with resistance training could have a positive effect on aging muscle mass and upper body strength compared to resistance training alone [69]. In agreement with these findings, the recent meta-analyses also showed that creatine supplementation leads to greater increases in muscle mass (SMD: 1.37 kg [95% CI = 0.97–1.76]) and leg muscle strength (SMD: 0.24 kg [95% CI = 0.05–0.43]) in participants with a mean age of 57–70 years [70]. The molecular mechanisms underlying the improved protein synthesis and muscle strength following creatine administration might be correlated with an increase in skeletal muscle phosphocreatine content and enhanced muscle glycogen storage through exercise [67]. Despite these promising results, it is worth to mention that the vast majority of these studies measured the impact of combined exercise interventions and creatine supplementation in the sarcopenic populations suffering from malnutrition [69].

2.2 Role of n-3 fatty acids in prevention and treatment of sarcopenia

Many nutrients also have anabolic effects on aging musculoskeletal health. There is growing evidence for an association between n-3 fatty acids intake alone or in combination of other nutrients and components of sarcopenia, including muscle mass, muscle strength, and physical performance [71, 72]. In this regard, the investigation of possible relationship between circulating *n*-3 FA levels and sarcopenia among 125 participants in Asian older adults indicated that subjects with low muscle strength had 32.4% lower serum *n*-3 concentrations ($P = 0.030$) than controls [73]. In addition, omega-3 fatty acids intake was lower in elderly sarcopenic patients than elderly subjects without sarcopenia [2.6 ± 1.0 vs. 3.0 ± 1.2 kcal/day, p = 0.046] [74].

Furthermore, the recent results of the Maastricht Sarcopenia Study also showed that sarcopenic older adults had a 10–18% lower intake of five nutrients (n-3 fatty acids, vitamin B_6, folic acid, vitamin E, magnesium) compared with non-sarcopenic older adults ($P < .05$) [55]. Similarly, prolonged supplementation with omega-3 fatty acids has been examined in older adults in order to improve the muscle protein synthetic response [75, 76], and importantly, the combined supplements providing high-quality proteins, leucine, vitamin D, and omega-3 fatty acids all together appear to be most favorable effects in the prevention of sarcopenia, while also being safe [77]. The positive effects of omega-3 fatty acids supplementation on muscle mass and function have also been identified by a systematic review and meta-analysis [72]. In addition, some studies specified that vitamin D supplementation combined with n-3 fatty acids, in particular EPA + DHA, may have favorable effect on physical function, muscle mass, and strength [77]. It is supposed that the anti-inflammatory effects of omega-3 fatty acids have an important role in the reduction in sarcopenia risk [78]. Nevertheless, the exact mechanisms by which n-3 fatty acids apply their beneficial effects on components of sarcopenia remain to be elucidated.

2.3 Role of vitamin D in prevention and treatment of sarcopenia

Among several nutrients, there has been increasing interest in the implications of vitamin D, either as single supplements or in combination with other supplements, for improving the physical function of older adults due to high prevalence of vitamin D deficiency [79]. A positive correlation between serum 25(OH)D concentration and muscle function has been shown [80]. The previous systematic reviews aimed at examining the benefits of vitamin D supplementation on sarcopenia in aging indicated the importance of considering baseline serum 25(OH)D concentrations in the response to supplementation [81]. While, concerning this issue, the recent meta-analysis of RCTs (2017) confirmed a slight improvement in the physical performance test following supplementation, no overall increase in handgrip strength was detected [82]. Nevertheless, this finding strengthens that vitamin D with a range of 800–1000 IU/day, but not necessarily at higher doses, has beneficial effect on muscle strength [77].

2.4 Role of gut microbiota in prevention and treatment of sarcopenia

Epidemiologic studies point out that altered gut microbiota structure according to diet, taking drugs, and other environmental factors across the lifespan result in different microbiota patterns, composition, and function in the elderly [83, 84]. The gut microbiota has the essential function maintaining some aspects of health [85]. Changing microbiota patterns are associated with significant changes in metabolic and physiologic regulation, and markers of inflammation that could result in age-related adverse health consequences [86, 87]. Recent researchers have postulated that gut microbiota composition may have a great relationship with age-related alterations in skeletal muscle function [87]. In this concern, experimental studies revealed that changes in the gut composition via probiotic/prebiotic administration could influence muscle function and inflammatory status [88–90]. Our recent meta-analysis emphasized that probiotic supplementation for more than 12 weeks has positive impact on the muscle strength. However, the clear mechanism underlying the positive effect of probiotic administration on muscle strength was not identified. The possible explanation for these findings may be related to reduced levels of IGF-1 (insulin-like growth factor 1) during lifetime [39, 91]. The beneficial probiotic effects on circulating inflammatory biomarkers could be another description [92].

2.5 Role of dietary quality in prevention of sarcopenia

Research on dietary quality and dietary patterns has recently been undertaken to better understand the effects of diet as a whole and its impact on aging health complication such as sarcopenia. Results of recent cross-sectional study in 250 menopausal women 45 years old or older found that Mediterranean dietary pattern has a favorable role in the prevention of sarcopenia [93]. Additionally, adherence to dietary pattern including "vegetables-fruits" was associated with lower odds of prevalent sarcopenia in Chinese older men [94]. Furthermore, it is shown that subjects with higher consumption of "snacks-drinks-milk products" score had lower odds of sarcopenia (OR = 0.41, 95% CI: 0.24–0.70, $P_{trend} < 0.001$) [94]. Interestingly, findings of recent cross-sectional study revealed that adherence to the Western dietary pattern, characterized by a high intake of sugar, soy, and fast foods, was not linked to sarcopenia (OR = 0.51; 95% CI: 0.21–1.24; $P_{trend} = 0.13$) [95]. The link between healthier diets and physical performance among older adults has been proposed [41]. However, there is not enough research evidence available in various communities to inform about the definitive decision on the specific food pattern for the prevention or treatment of sarcopenia.

3. Conclusion

Age-related sarcopenia is a phenomenon with significant disability among the elderly. This condition is one of the most important public health problems among the healthy community. While there are the various notable bodies of research in order to define sarcopenia, the diversity in the cutoffs of the sarcopenia's characterization revealed the needs for more research to define accurate reference values in different nations and countries around the world. On the other hand, one of the main controversial topics in evaluating the influence of nutrition on age-related sarcopenia is related to various definitions of sarcopenia in different nations and countries. In addition, due to the lack of a valid biomarker for the detection of sarcopenia, the exact mechanism underlying beneficial effect of numerous nutritional factors on components of sarcopenia remains unknown. Furthermore, there is not enough research evidence available in various communities to inform about the definitive decision on the food for the prevention or treatment of sarcopenia. The other limitation of included studies in this review was connected to absence of information about dietary intakes and serum concentrations of many micronutrients in older adults. So, considering the biochemical levels and dietary intakes of micronutrients in future studies is recommended. Finally, further studies are needed to investigate the interaction effect of modifiable risk factors, in particularly nutrition over time based in the near future.

Overall, present findings from the scientific literature specified that the combined nutritional supplements, such as vitamin D, n-3 fatty acids, and creatine along with resistance training could have better improvement in aging muscle mass and upper body strength compared with each alone. This effect particularly was shown in subjects with low serum vitamin D concentrations. In addition, it seems that the beneficial effect of probiotic/prebiotic administration also depends on changed gut microbiota composition. It is worth to mention that adherence to healthy dietary pattern with high quality including vegetables and fruits may lead to lower odds of sarcopenia.

Conflict of interest

None.

Author details

Nafiseh Shokri-Mashhadi
Food Security Research Center and Department of Clinical Nutrition, School of Nutrition and Food Science, Isfahan University of Medical Sciences, Isfahan, Iran

*Address all correspondence to: nafiseh.shokri@yahoo.com

References

[1] Burch JB et al. Advances in geroscience: Impact on healthspan and chronic disease. Journals of Gerontology Series A: Biomedical Sciences and Medical Sciences. 2014;**69**(Suppl_1):S1-S3

[2] Nargund G. Declining birth rate in Developed Countries: A radical policy re-think is required. Facts, Views & Vision in ObGyn. 2009;**1**(3):191-193

[3] Castrejón-Pérez RC et al. Frailty, diabetes, and the convergence of chronic disease in an age-related condition: A population-based nationwide cross-sectional analysis of the Mexican nutrition and health survey. Aging Clinical and Experimental Research. 2018;**30**(8):935-941

[4] Rosenberg IH. Sarcopenia: Origins and clinical relevance. The Journal of Nutrition. 1997;**127**(5):990S-991S

[5] Rosenberg IH. Summary comments. The American Journal of Clinical Nutrition. 1989;**50**(5):1231-1233

[6] Reiss J et al. Consequences of applying the new EWGSOP2 guideline instead of the former EWGSOP guideline for sarcopenia case finding in older patients. Age and Ageing. 2019;**48**(5):719-724

[7] Cruz-Jentoft AJ et al. Sarcopenia: European consensus on definition and diagnosisReport of the European Working Group on Sarcopenia in Older PeopleA. J. Cruz-Gentoft et al. Age and Ageing. 2010;**39**(4):412-423

[8] Lang T et al. Sarcopenia: Etiology, clinical consequences, intervention, and assessment. Osteoporosis International. 2010;**21**(4):543-559

[9] Cruz-Jentoft A. European Working Group on Sarcopenia in Older People: Sarcopenia: European consensus on definition and diagnosis. Report of the European Working Group on Sarcopenia in Older People. Age and Ageing. 2010;**39**:412-423

[10] Tosato M et al. Measurement of muscle mass in sarcopenia: From imaging to biochemical markers. Aging Clinical and Experimental Research. 2017;**29**(1):19-27

[11] Ida S et al. Sarcopenia is a predictor of postoperative respiratory complications in patients with esophageal cancer. Annals of Surgical Oncology. 2015;**22**(13):4432-4437

[12] Heymsfield SB et al. Assessing skeletal muscle mass: Historical overview and state of the art. Journal of Cachexia, Sarcopenia and Muscle. 2014;**5**(1):9-18

[13] Malafarina V et al. Sarcopenia in the elderly: Diagnosis, physiopathology and treatment. Maturitas. 2012;**71**(2):109-114

[14] Baumgartner RN et al. Predictors of skeletal muscle mass in elderly men and women. Mechanisms of Ageing and Development. 1999;**107**(2):123-136

[15] Newman AB et al. Strength and muscle quality in a well-functioning cohort of older adults: The Health, Aging and Body Composition Study. Journal of the American Geriatrics Society. 2003;**51**(3):323-330

[16] Assantachai P et al. Cut-off points of quadriceps strength, declines and relationships of sarcopenia-related variables among T hai community-dwelling older adults. Geriatrics & Gerontology International. 2014;**14**:61-68

[17] Wilson D et al. Frailty and sarcopenia: The potential role of an aged immune system. Ageing Research Reviews. 2017;**36**:1-10

[18] Ferrucci L, Fabbri E. Inflammageing: Chronic inflammation in ageing, cardiovascular disease, and frailty. Nature Reviews Cardiology. 2018;**15**(9):1

[19] Ilia S. Stop Aging Disease! ICAD 2014. Aging and Disease. 2015;**6**(2):76

[20] Deleidi M, Jäggle M, Rubino G. Immune aging, dysmetabolism, and inflammation in neurological diseases. Frontiers in Neuroscience. 2015;**9**:172

[21] Londhe P, Guttridge DC. Inflammation induced loss of skeletal muscle. Bone. 2015;**80**:131-142

[22] Bar-Shai M et al. The effect of hindlimb immobilization on acid phosphatase, metalloproteinases and nuclear factor-κB in muscles of young and old rats. Mechanisms of Ageing and Development. 2005;**126**(2):289-297

[23] Lin H et al. Whole blood gene expression and interleukin-6 levels. Genomics. 2014;**104**(6):490-495

[24] Paolisso G et al. Advancing age and insulin resistance: Role of plasma tumor necrosis factor-α. American Journal of Physiology-Endocrinology And Metabolism. 1998;**275**(2):E294-E299

[25] Shokri-Mashhadi N et al. Association of circulating C-reactive protein and high-sensitivity C-reactive protein with components of sarcopenia: A systematic review and meta-analysis of observational studies. Experimental Gerontology. 2021;**150**:111330

[26] Hida T et al. Sarcopenia and physical function are associated with inflammation and arteriosclerosis in community-dwelling people: The Yakumo study. Modern Rheumatology. 2018;**28**(2):345-350

[27] Ryan AS. Insulin resistance with aging. Sports Medicine. 2000;**30**(5): 327-346

[28] Cleasby ME, Jamieson PM, Atherton PJ. Insulin resistance and sarcopenia: Mechanistic links between common co-morbidities. Journal of Endocrinology. 2016;**229**(2):R67-R81

[29] Kim S-H, Kwon HS, Hwang H-J. White blood cell counts, insulin resistance, vitamin D levels and sarcopenia in Korean elderly men. Scandinavian Journal of Clinical and Laboratory Investigation. 2017;**77**(3):228-233

[30] Gorshunova N, Medvedev N. Significance of insulin resistance in the pathogenesis of sarcopenia and chronic heart failure in elderly hypertensive patients. Advances in Gerontology—Uspekhi Gerontologii. 2016;**29**(2):324-328

[31] Johannsen DL et al. Ectopic lipid accumulation and reduced glucose tolerance in elderly adults are accompanied by altered skeletal muscle mitochondrial activity. The Journal of Clinical Endocrinology & Metabolism. 2012;**97**(1):242-250

[32] Stuart CA et al. Slow-twitch fiber proportion in skeletal muscle correlates with insulin responsiveness. The Journal of Clinical Endocrinology & Metabolism. 2013;**98**(5):2027-2036

[33] Yarasheski K et al. Serum myostatin-immunoreactive protein is increased in 60-92 year old women and men with muscle wasting. Journal of Nutrition Health and Aging. 2002;**6**(5):343-348

[34] Bonala S et al. Myostatin induces insulin resistance via Casitas B-lineage lymphoma b (Cblb)-mediated degradation of insulin receptor substrate 1 (IRS1) in response to high calorie diet intake. The Journal of Biological Chemistry. 2016;**291**(27):14392

[35] Dagdeviren S et al. IL-10 prevents aging-associated inflammation and insulin resistance in skeletal muscle. The FASEB Journal. 2016;**31**(2):701-710

[36] Vitale G, Cesari M, Mari D. Aging of the endocrine system and its potential impact on sarcopenia. European Journal of Internal Medicine. 2016;**35**:10-15

[37] Chahal H, Drake W. The endocrine system and ageing. The Journal of Pathology: A Journal of the Pathological Society of Great Britain and Ireland. 2007;**211**(2):173-180

[38] Sattler FR. Growth hormone in the aging male. Best Practice & Research Clinical Endocrinology & Metabolism. 2013;**27**(4):541-555

[39] Van Nieuwpoort C et al. The relationship between serum IGF-1, handgrip strength, physical performance and falls in elderly men and women. European Journal of Endocrinology. 2018;**179**(2):EJE-18-0076

[40] Bosaeus I, Rothenberg E. Nutrition and physical activity for the prevention and treatment of age-related sarcopenia. Proceedings of the Nutrition Society. 2015;**75**(2):174-180

[41] Bloom I et al. Diet quality and sarcopenia in older adults: A systematic review. Nutrients. 2018;**10**(3):308

[42] Hayashi T et al. Association between sarcopenia and depressive mood in urban-dwelling older adults: A cross-sectional study. Geriatrics & Gerontology International. 2019;**19**(6):508-512

[43] Gruber ES et al. Sarcopenia and sarcopenic obesity are independent adverse prognostic factors in resectable pancreatic ductal adenocarcinoma. PLoS One. 2019;**14**(5):e0215915

[44] Fiatarone MA et al. The Boston FICSIT study: The effects of resistance training and nutritional supplementation on physical frailty in the oldest old. Journal of the American Geriatrics Society. 1993;**41**(3):333-337

[45] De Jong N et al. Dietary supplements and physical exercise affecting bone and body composition in frail elderly persons. American Journal of Public Health. 2000;**90**(6):947

[46] Chang K-V et al. Association between sarcopenia and cognitive impairment: A systematic review and meta-analysis. Journal of the American Medical Directors Association. 2016;**17**(12):1164. e7-1164. e15

[47] Laviano A, Gori C, Rianda S. Sarcopenia and nutrition. Advances in Food and Nutrition Research. 2014;**71**:101-136

[48] Walston JD. Sarcopenia in older adults. Current Opinion in Rheumatology. 2012;**24**(6):623

[49] Agarwal E et al. Malnutrition in the elderly: A narrative review. Maturitas. 2013;**76**(4):296-302

[50] Eglseer D, Eminovic S, Lohrmann C. Association between sarcopenia and nutritional status in older adults: A systematic literature review. Journal of Gerontological Nursing. 2016;**42**(7):33-41

[51] Morley JE et al. Nutritional recommendations for the management of sarcopenia. Journal of the American

Medical Directors Association. 2010;**11**(6):391-396

[52] Seo MH et al. The association between daily calcium intake and sarcopenia in older, non-obese Korean adults: The fourth Korea National Health and Nutrition Examination Survey (KNHANES IV) 2009. Endocrine Journal. 2013;**60**(5):679-686

[53] Bauer J et al. Evidence-based recommendations for optimal dietary protein intake in older people: A position paper from the PROT-AGE study group. Journal of the American Medical Directors Association. 2013;**14**(8):542-559

[54] Paddon-Jones D et al. Role of dietary protein in the sarcopenia of aging. The American Journal of Clinical Nutrition. 2008;**87**(5):1562S-1566S

[55] ter Borg S et al. Differences in nutrient intake and biochemical nutrient status between sarcopenic and nonsarcopenic older adults—results from the Maastricht Sarcopenia Study. Journal of the American Medical Directors Association. 2016;**17**(5):393-401

[56] Pasiakos SM et al. Acute Energy Deprivation Affects Skeletal Muscle Protein Synthesis and Associated Intracellular Signaling Proteins in Physically Active Adults, 2. The Journal of Nutrition. 2010;**140**(4):745-751

[57] Joint WHO. FAO/UNU expert consultation. Protein and amino acid requirements in human nutrition. World Health Organanization Technical Report Series. Vol. 935. 2007. pp. 1-265

[58] Volpi E et al. Is the optimal level of protein intake for older adults greater than the recommended dietary allowance? Journals of Gerontology Series A: Biomedical Sciences and Medical Sciences. 2013;**68**(6):677-681

[59] Trappe T et al. Influence of concurrent exercise or nutrition countermeasures on thigh and calf muscle size and function during 60 days of bed rest in women. Acta Physiologica. 2007;**191**(2):147-159

[60] Beasley JM, Shikany JM, Thomson CA. The role of dietary protein intake in the prevention of sarcopenia of aging. Nutrition in Clinical Practice. 2013;**28**(6):684-690

[61] van Loon LJ. Leucine as a pharmaconutrient in health and disease. Current Opinion in Clinical Nutrition & Metabolic Care. 2012;**15**(1):71-77

[62] Englund DA et al. Nutritional supplementation with physical activity improves muscle composition in mobility-limited older adults, the VIVE2 study: A randomized, double-blind, placebo-controlled trial. The Journals of Gerontology: Series A. 2017;**73**(1):95-101

[63] Wall BT, Van Loon LJ. Nutritional strategies to attenuate muscle disuse atrophy. Nutrition Reviews. 2013;**71**(4):195-208

[64] Tieland M et al. The impact of dietary protein or amino acid supplementation on muscle mass and strength in elderly people: Individual participant data and meta-analysis of rct's. The Journal of Nutrition, Health & Aging. 2017;**21**(9):994-1001

[65] Greenhaff PL. The creatine-phosphocreatine system: There's more than one song in its repertoire. The Journal of Physiology. 2001;**537**(Pt 3):657

[66] Riesberg LA et al. Beyond muscles: The untapped potential of creatine.

International Immunopharmacology. 2016;**37**:31-42

[67] Tarnopolsky MA, Safdar A. The potential benefits of creatine and conjugated linoleic acid as adjuncts to resistance training in older adults. Applied Physiology, Nutrition, and Metabolism. 2008;**33**(1):213-227

[68] Beaudart C et al. Nutrition and physical activity in the prevention and treatment of sarcopenia: Systematic review. Osteoporosis International. 2017;**28**(6):1817-1833

[69] Candow DG, Chilibeck PD, Forbes SC. Creatine supplementation and aging musculoskeletal health. Endocrine. 2014;**45**(3):354-361

[70] Chilibeck PD et al. Effect of creatine supplementation during resistance training on lean tissue mass and muscular strength in older adults: A meta-analysis. Open access Journal of Sports Medicine. 2017;**8**:213

[71] Santiago EC et al. Comparison of calorie and nutrient intake among elderly with and without sarcopenia: A systematic review and meta-analysis. Nutrition Reviews. 2021;**79**(12):1338-1352

[72] Bird JK et al. The effect of long chain omega-3 polyunsaturated fatty acids on muscle mass and function in sarcopenia: A scoping systematic review and meta-analysis. Clinical Nutrition ESPEN. 2021;**46**:73-86

[73] Jang I-Y et al. Lower Serum n-3 Fatty Acid Level in Older Adults with Sarcopenia. Nutrients. 2020;**12**(10):2959

[74] Okamura T et al. Reduced dietary omega-3 fatty acids intake is associated with sarcopenia in elderly patients with type 2 diabetes: A cross-sectional study of KAMOGAWA-DM cohort study. Journal of Clinical Biochemistry and Nutrition. 2020;**66**(3):19-85

[75] Hutchins-Wiese H et al. The impact of supplemental n-3 long chain polyunsaturated fatty acids and dietary antioxidants on physical performance in postmenopausal women. The Journal of Nutrition, Health & Aging. 2013;**17**(1):76-80

[76] Smith GI et al. Fish oil–derived n− 3 PUFA therapy increases muscle mass and function in healthy older adults. The American Journal of Clinical Nutrition. 2015;**102**(1):115-122

[77] Tessier A-J, Chevalier S. An update on protein, leucine, omega-3 fatty acids, and vitamin D in the prevention and treatment of sarcopenia and functional decline. Nutrients. 2018;**10**(8):1099

[78] Gray SR, Mittendorfer B. Fish oil-derived n-3 polyunsaturated fatty acids for the prevention and treatment of sarcopenia. Current Opinion in Clinical Nutrition & Metabolic Care. 2018;**21**(2):104-109

[79] Lips P, van Schoor N. Worldwide Vitamin D Status, in Vitamin D (Third Edition). Amsterdam, Netherlands: Elsevier; 2011. pp. 947-963

[80] Okazaki R et al. Assessment criteria for vitamin D deficiency/insufficiency in Japan: Proposal by an expert panel supported by the Research Program of Intractable Diseases, Ministry of Health, Labour and Welfare, Japan, the Japanese Society for Bone and Mineral Research and the Japan Endocrine Society [Opinion]. Journal of Bone and Mineral Metabolism. 2017;**35**(1):1-5

[81] Annweiler C et al. Vitamin D-related changes in physical performance:

A systematic review. The Journal of Nutrition, Health & Aging. 2009;**13**(10):893-898

[82] Rosendahl-Riise H et al. Vitamin D supplementation and its influence on muscle strength and mobility in community-dwelling older persons: A systematic review and meta-analysis. Journal of Human Nutrition and Dietetics. 2017;**30**(1):3-15

[83] Lakshminarayanan B et al. Compositional dynamics of the human intestinal microbiota with aging: Implications for health. The Journal of Nutrition, Health & Aging. 2014;**18**(9):773-786

[84] Siddharth J et al. Aging and sarcopenia associate with specific interactions between gut microbes, serum biomarkers and host physiology in rats. Aging (Albany NY). 2017;**9**(7):1698

[85] Tiihonen K, Ouwehand AC, Rautonen N. Human intestinal microbiota and healthy ageing. Ageing Research Reviews. 2010;**9**(2):107-116

[86] Ticinesi A et al. Aging gut microbiota at the cross-road between nutrition, physical frailty, and sarcopenia: Is there a gut–muscle axis? Nutrients. 2017;**9**(12):1303

[87] Ticinesi A et al. Gut microbiota, muscle mass and function in aging: A focus on physical frailty and sarcopenia. Nutrients. 2019;**11**(7):1633

[88] Iolascon G et al. Pharmacological therapy of sarcopenia: Past, present and future. Clinical Cases in Mineral & Bone Metabolism. 2018;**15**(3):407-415

[89] Ni Y et al. Lactobacillus and Bifidobacterium improves physiological function and cognitive ability in aged mice by the regulation of gut microbiota. Molecular Nutrition & Food Research. 2019;**63**(22):1900603

[90] Lahiri S et al. The gut microbiota influences skeletal muscle mass and function in mice. Science Translational Medicine. 2019;**11**(502):eaan5662

[91] Barbieri M et al. Chronic inflammation and the effect of IGF-I on muscle strength and power in older persons. American Journal of Physiology-Endocrinology and Metabolism. 2003;**284**(3):E481-E487

[92] Kazemi A et al. Effect of probiotic and synbiotic supplementation on inflammatory markers in health and disease status: A systematic review and meta-analysis of clinical trials. Clinical Nutrition. 2020;**39**(3):789-819

[93] Mohseni R et al. Relationship between major dietary patterns and sarcopenia among menopausal women. Aging Clinical and Experimental Research. 2017;**29**(6):1241-1248

[94] Chan R, Leung J, Woo J. A prospective cohort study to examine the association between dietary patterns and sarcopenia in Chinese community-dwelling older people in Hong Kong. Journal of the American Medical Directors Association. 2016;**17**(4):336-342

[95] Hashemi R et al. Diet and its relationship to sarcopenia in community dwelling Iranian elderly: A cross sectional study. Nutrition. 2015;**31**(1):97-104

Chapter 7

Perspective Chapter: Nutraceuticals as a Therapeutic Promise in Healthy Aging and Neurocognitive Disorders

Abhishek Ramesh and Debanjan Banerjee

Abstract

The world is facing a rapid population ageing. Noncommunicable disorders (NCDs) form the bulk of present-day morbidity. Besides dealing with neurodegeneration and neurocognitive disorders, modern-day therapeutics have also geared toward healthy ageing and preventive approaches. Several chemical substances belonging to classes of natural dietary origin display protective properties against some age related diseases, including neurodegenerative ones. These compounds, known as nutraceuticals, differ structurally, acting on different pathways. There has been a paradigm shift in the understanding of dementias toward neuroinflammation, oxidative stress, immunomodulation, and gut-brain axis dysregulation. This offers promise for the nutraceuticals as a novel approach in the field of neurocognitive disorders and healthy ageing. However, the collective evidence is still evolving and as of yet not robust enough for nutraceuticals to be a part of clinical guidelines. The other caveats are lack of subjective understanding of use, and individual constituents of a product showing differential effects, which lead to ambiguous outcomes in clinical trials. This chapter critically looks at the role of various nutraceuticals in promoting healthy aging and management of neurodegenerative conditions (especially Alzheimer's disease). The evidence so far is highlighted with the challenges in their use and future directions of research.

Keywords: neurocognition, neurocognitive disorders, healthy aging, nutraceuticals, dietary natural products, neuroprotection, dementia

1. Introduction

Aging can be defined as the time-related deterioration of the physiological functions necessary for survival and fertility. It affects all the individuals of a species [1]. Age is a major risk factor for numerous illnesses, such as diabetes and cancer, various degenerative diseases, including Alzheimer's disease (AD), Huntington's disease (HD), Parkinson's disease (PDs), and various other neurocognitive disorders (NCDs) [2]. However, genetics, lifestyle patterns, environment, and ecology play an equal or perhaps more important role in these diseases. Different biological theories have been put forward to explain the aging phenomena. Some of these are oxidative damage theory, general wear and tear theory, genetic instability, telomere shortening, mitochondrial genome damage, genetic program theory, etc. [1, 3–10].

Cognition is the higher order brain function that alters with advancing age, which, in turn, influences the quality of life of an individual [11]. Cognitive aging is governed by the interplay of multiple factors, including lifestyle, diet, nutrition, endocrine and genetic parameters, oxidative damage, neurotoxic exposures, and medical and surgical interventions for disease [12, 13]. Nutritional status plays a critical role in the cognitive abilities of an individual. It is a modifier of cognitive aging. Studies have shown that nutritional imbalance adversely affects the structural and functional integrity of the brain critically impacting the cognitive capacities and process of aging [14].

Older people are at risk for various micronutrient deficiencies due to social, physical, economic, and emotional factors. The development of effective nutritional interventions for promoting healthy aging and preventing and treating NCDs is an emerging and challenging area of biomedical research [13].

The term "nutraceutical" was originally defined by Stephen L. DeFelice, as a combination of terms *"nutrition and pharmaceutical* [15]." As per the European Nutraceutical Association, they are defined as *"naturally derived bioactive compounds that are found in foods, dietary supplements, and herbal products, and have health-promoting, disease-preventing, or medicinal properties* [16]." On the other hand, "nutritional supplements" are nutritional compounds that supplement one's diet by increasing total daily intake [17]. Nutraceuticals are intended to affect the structure and function of the body; however, they do not undergo premarket approval. These are perceived as safe and less likely to have adverse effects [18]. Nutraceutical categories include dietary supplements (e.g., vitamins, minerals, coenzyme Q, carnitine, and botanicals such as ginseng and ginkgo biloba), medicinal foods (e.g., transgenic plants), and functional foods (e.g., oats, bran, omega-3 fatty acids, and plant sterols) [15, 19].

"Nutritional psychiatry" is a distinct field of psychiatry that studies the role and impact of diet and various nutraceuticals in the treatment and prevention of a range of psychiatric disorders, including neurocognitive disorders (NCDs) [20–22].

The role of nutraceuticals in noncommunicable diseases and healthy aging has been increasingly studied. Though the evidence base for their use in neurocognitive disorders has been increasing, guidelines regulating their use, safety, adverse effects, and efficacy in clinical settings are ambiguous and limited. There is a general tendency to accept "nutraceutical products" as a part of nutritional supplements in healthy aging with an "assumption" of their safety; however, more research is needed in the field [17, 18]. The ambiguity in evidence makes it challenging for clinicians working in the field of neuropsychiatry to take a clear stand related to their use and effectiveness. Keeping this in background, this chapter provides an overview of various nutraceuticals used in healthy aging and neurocognitive disorders, summarizes the available evidence base for the same, discusses the possible mechanisms of action, and outlines the challenges involved in their clinical use. This chapter is expected to stimulate thoughts and further research into this promising area that can offer viable solutions in the field of neurocognition.

2. Types of nutraceuticals that have been studied in NCDs and healthy aging

2.1 Mechanism of action: how do nutraceuticals intervene?

The majority of nutraceuticals act as antioxidant agents; few of them are anti-inflammatory, anticarcinogenic, and antiangiogenic agents (**Table 1**) [13, 35]. The

Class of nutraceuticals	Mechanism of action	Examples and diet sources
Antioxidants [23]	Inhibit the formation of free radicals by breaking the chain reaction or reduce the concentration of free radicals by donating hydrogen and electron	Vitamin A, E, C, Polyphenols, Beta carotene (green leafy vegetables and citrus fruits)
Plant polyphenols and catechins [24]	Antioxidant, Anti-inflammatory, Anticancer	Turmeric, green tea, Grapeseed (fruits, vegetables, legumes, cereals, and beverages)
Carotenoids [25]	Anticancer, Antioxidant, Cell growth regulation, modulation of gene expression, and immune response	Lutein, zeaxanthin, and lycopene, (green leafy vegetables, spinach, carrots, and apricots)
Plant stanols/sterols (Phytosterols) [26]	Reduce cholesterol absorption, anti-inflammatory, antineoplastic, and immunomodulating	Sitosterol, stigmasterol, campesterol, (vegetables, nuts, fruits, and seeds)
B vitamins [27]	One carbon metabolism, Methylation reactions	Vitamin B6, B9, B12
Calcium and vitamin D [28]	Bone metabolism, antineoplastic	Spinach, soybeans, fish
Omega-3 fatty acids [29]	Anti-inflammatory, Reduce blood triglyceride levels	Eicosapentaenoic acid (EPA), docosahexaenoic acid (DHA), (fish oil, plants, flaxseed)
Prebiotics and probiotics [30]	Role in innate immunity, intestinal barrier function	Lactobacillus and Bifidobacterium family
Zinc [31]	DNA synthesis, cell proliferation, and differentiation	Whole grain, legumes, meat, egg, sea fish
Coenzyme Q10 [28]	Aerobic respiration, generation of ATP	
Ginkgo biloba [32]	Improves function of nerve cells, platelets, and antioxidant	
Vaccinium corymbosum (blueberry) [28]	Antioxidant,	blueberry
Cranberry (Vaccinium oxycoccos) and oregano (Origanum vulgare) [33]	Antimicrobial, antiviral, antimutagenic, antiangiogenic, and antioxidant	
Nectarine and acai fruits [28]	Antioxidant	
Rosa damascena	Antiepileptic, anti-amyloid	Rose oil
Cocoa polyphenols [28]	Antioxidant, altering chromatin structure	Cocoa powder
Quercetin and tannic acid [34]	Antiamyloid, antineoplastic, antioxidant	Fruits and vegetables
Caffeic acid and rosmarinic acid	Anticarcinogenic, antirheumatic, and anti-inflammatory	Fruits, vegetables, and herbs
Spermidine	Enhance autophagy	Citrus fruits, soybean

Table 1.
Various nutraceuticals (and their sources) that have been studied in healthy aging and NCDs.

various ways in which they act on cognitive processes and aging are depicted in **Figure 1**. However, these are only basics, and further research is necessary to elucidate the deeper underlying mechanisms.

2.1.1 Effects of nutraceuticals in cognitive aging and progression to neurodegenerative disorders

Cognitive changes associated with normal aging when accelerated result in mild cognitive impairment (MCI), characterized by structural changes in the brain such as amyloid plaque deposition, demyelination, and neurodegeneration. MCI increases the risk for developing major neurocognitive disorders through increased pathology, which results in marked cognitive impairment. Gene expression that has been altered with concomitant oxidative stress causes DNA damage and protein aggregation, which leads to MCI and dementia. Nutraceuticals of plant and animal origin help in the attainment of healthy aging and prevention and slow down the neurodegeneration process with increased longevity and preservation of cognitive abilities [36, 37]. Nutraceuticals have the potential to reverse structural changes in the brain, prevent DNA damage, and slow down protein aggregations promoting healthy aging as well as preventing or delaying the onset of MCI and dementia [13, 35, 38, 39]. Their effects on the cognitive changes in the pathophysiological spectrum are highlighted in **Figure 2**.

Both *in vivo* animal models and human studies in aging have shown that various nutraceuticals have a beneficial role in the promotion of positive mental health and well-being in aging, prevention of cognitive decline and eventually dementia, as well as slowing down the benign cognitive decline associated with normal aging [40–42]. Few nutraceuticals that were found to be useful in this regard are:

Brahmi herb (Bacopa monnieri): enhances cognitive performance in attention and logical memory domains and prevents and improves depressive symptoms.

Ashwagandha (Withania somnifera): enhances memory and sleep in aging and improves attention, executive functions, and information processing.

Turmeric (Curcuma longa): increases brain-derived neurotrophic factor (BDNF), prevents AD and depression.

Garlic (Allium sativum): reverses the levels of stress-related hormones and improves learning and memory.

Pumpkin seeds (Cucurbita maxima): improves memory and reduces depression [40].

Other nutraceuticals, including multivitamins, minerals such as zinc, selenium, and magnesium, fish oils, etc., also help in the improvement of cognitive functions in various domains [40, 43–47].

2.1.2 Role of nutraceuticals in other neurocognitive disorders

Most studies on the nutraceuticals' efficacy on neurocognitive disorders have focused on Alzheimer's disease. However, few studies have looked into the role of nutraceuticals in other neurocognitive disorders as well [39]. These studies are less robust and ambiguous in conclusive clinical implications.

In Parkinson's disease, nutraceuticals are found to be beneficial either by reducing the dose of L-dopa required or by acting independently, thus reducing the symptom severity [48]. *In vivo* studies have shown that vitamin B complex,

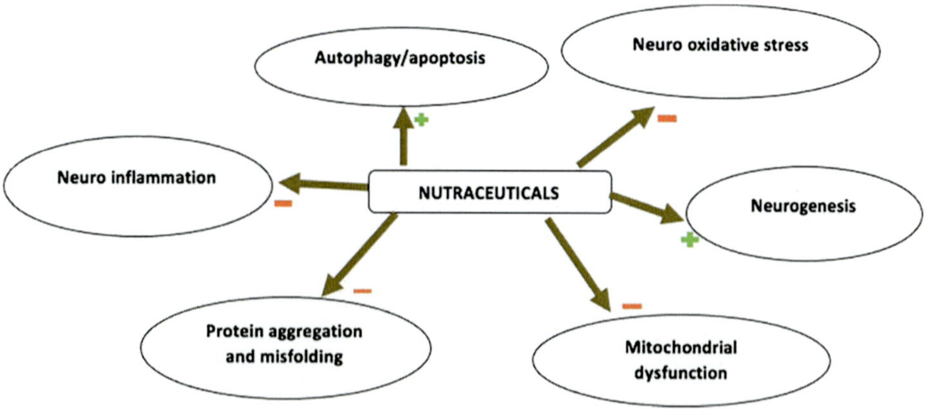

Figure 1.
Mechanisms in which nutraceuticals act on cognition and neurocognitive disorders [35].

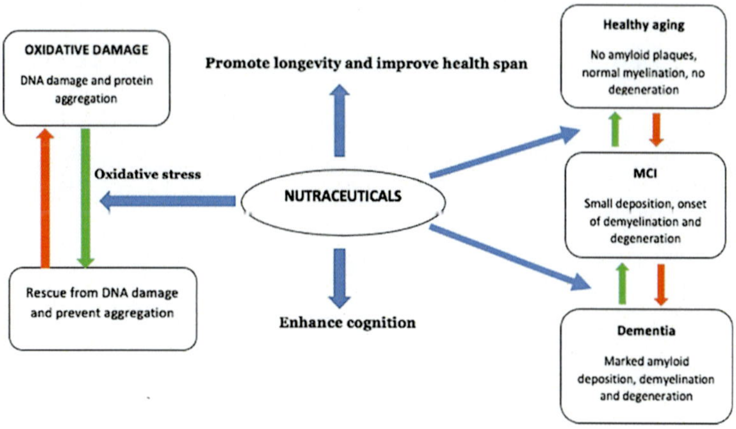

Figure 2.
Effect of nutraceuticals in mild cognitive impairment, neurocognitive disorders, and healthy aging.

vitamin D, creatine, fish oils, curcuminoids, mucuna seed powder extract, resveratrol, quercetin, Ginkgo biloba, etc., are beneficial in reducing the severity of motor symptoms, preventing the nonmotor symptoms and cognitive symptoms associated with PD [49, 50].

In vascular dementia (VD), the B vitamin complexes especially vitamins B6, B9, and B12 are found to be useful in preventing its occurrence [51]. Various Chinese herbal preparations, such as Ginkgo, Huperzia, curcumins, Ginseng, Brahmi, saffron, green tea, etc., found to be helpful as adjuvants for the pharmacological treatment of cognitive decline in VD [52]. The complex herbal formulations that include these herbal products in various combinations were found to be superior to the individual preparation [53, 54].

In patients with stroke and post-stroke sequelae, nutraceuticals are found to be clinically beneficial at various stages. They reduce the risk of occurrence of stroke and can be used as prophylactic agents to promote ischemic tolerance to delay, prevent, or postpone the occurrence or reoccurrence of stroke. They can also be used as adjunct therapeutic agents to minimize secondary brain damage in the case of acute stroke [55, 56]. Clinical studies have shown that vitamin B complex, vitamin E, magnesium, omega-3 fatty acids, polyphenols, and clinical studies have shown that coenzyme Q10, cystine, L-glutamate, retinoic acid, capsaicin, and vitamin D3 are useful as prophylactic agents. Nutraceuticals, including vitamin cocktail, minerals such as zinc and selenium, and curcumin, are used as therapeutic adjuvant agents in acute stroke for early recovery and prevention of complications [51, 56].

In Huntington's disease (HD), there are very few nutraceutical compounds that are found to be helpful. These include amino-oxy acetic acid (AOAA), levocarnitine [57], curcumin, taurine, resveratrol, anthocyanins, and quercetin [58]. Souvenaid™, a medical food composed of uridine monophosphate, DHA, choline, EPA, selenium, folic acid, phospholipids, and B vitamins has been found to have a significant positive impact on the behavioral symptomatology and theory of mind (ToM) skills in patients with frontotemporal dementia (FTD) [59].

2.1.3 Molecular mechanism of action of nutraceuticals in invertebrate models

Age is the major risk factor for various neurocognitive disorders [2]. There has been significant progress in elucidating the molecular mechanisms of aging [60, 61]. A number of genetic factors called longevity-related genes have been identified to modulate lifespan and health span in model organisms ranging from yeast, worms, flies, and rodents [62]. These genes fall into three nutrient sensing pathways:

- Target of rapamycin (TOR): sense cellular amino acid levels

- Insulin/IGF-1 like signaling (IIS): sense glucose levels

- Sirtuin pathway: sense NAD+ or NAD+/NADH levels

Nutraceuticals bind to the proteins that are translated from these genes, which will either inhibit or stimulate the further downward molecular pathway, leading finally to longevity and increased health span (**Figure 3**).

2.1.4 Interaction between nutraceuticals and the gut microbiota

The gut microbiota is a collection of colonies of multiple microbes that reside in the body and live in a symbiotic relationship with their host [63]. The brain-gut-microbiota axis comprises a part of this microbiota that is an extensive communication network between the brain [64] and gut. This axis plays an important role in the emotional and cognitive development of an individual, and any dysbiosis in this axis will lead to the occurrence of neuropsychiatric illnesses [65, 66]. Recent studies have shown the interaction between hypothalamo-pituitary–adrenal (HPA) axis and brain-gut-microbiota axis in the causation of psychiatric disorders [63].

Probiotics are various bacterial strains that exert beneficial effects through the number of ways such as antimicrobial effects, modulating the host's immune response, enhancing the functioning of epithelial barrier [63, 67]. The recent studies at the preliminary stage have shown that nutraceuticals, including prebiotics (fructo-oligosaccharides, xylo-oligosaccharides, and inulins), anthraquinones, phytoestrogens, polyphenols, amino acids, vitamins, and omega-3 fatty acids, can interact with

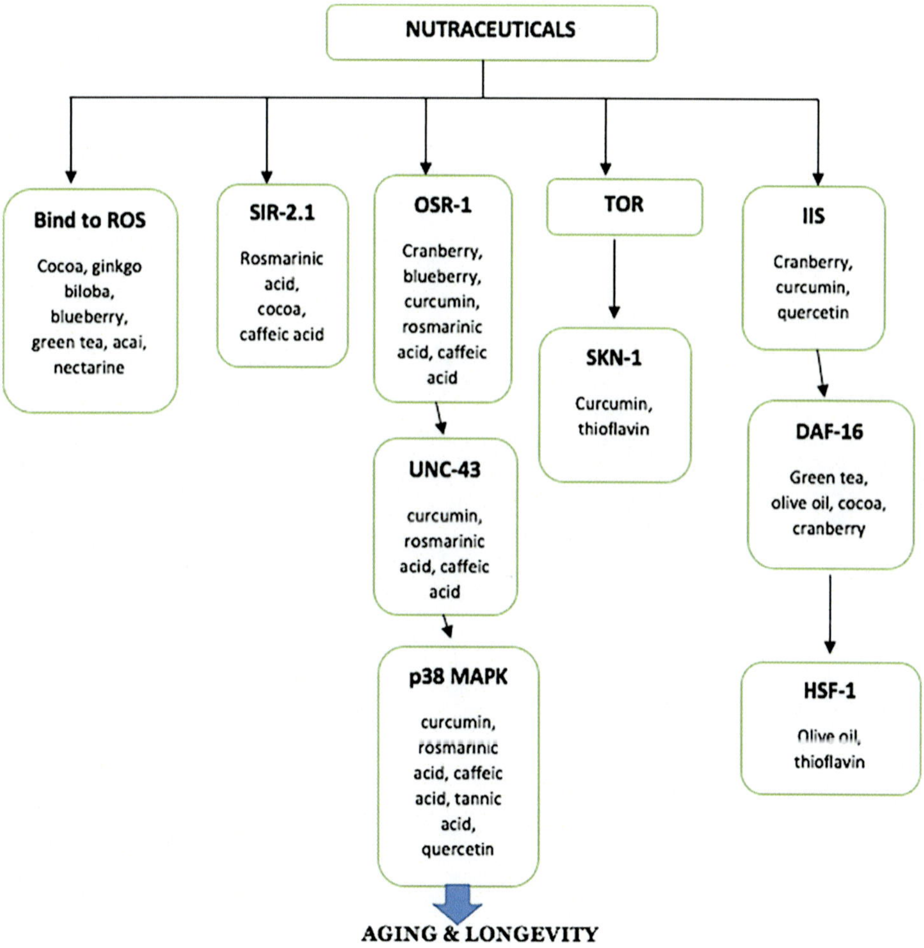

Figure 3.
Schematic representation of nutrient signaling, and stress response pathways associated with aging and longevity in C. elegans and D. melanogaster [62]. ROS: Reactive oxygen species, SIR: Sirtuin, OSR: Osmotic stress resistant, MAPK: Mitogen activated protein kinase, UNC: Calcium/calmodulin dependent protein kinase, TOR: Target of rapamycin, SKN: Gene for protein skinhead-1, IIS: Insulin/IGF-1 like signaling, DAF: Gene for FOXO protein, HSF: Heat shock transcription factor.

gut microbiota, often improving the diversity of gut microbiota, regulating immune function of the host, and improving the integrity of the intestinal barrier, which may have a beneficial role in the prevention and treatment of various neuropsychiatric and neurocognitive disorders [68–71].

3. Evidence based on nutraceuticals in neurocognitive disorders and healthy aging

There are a number of studies that have investigated the efficacy of nutraceuticals in the prevention and treatment of neurocognitive disorders. These studies vary from each other in terms of methodology, sampling size and strategies, study design, duration of treatment, and selection and doses of various nutraceuticals [72]. The results of all these studies are largely mixed. Therefore, these studies need to be replicated in larger

Study	Study type	Sample characteristics	Intervention	Study duration	Results
de Jager et al. [74]	Double blind single-centre randomized controlled trial	Diagnosis-MCI n = 266 (intervention = 133, control = 133) mean age = 76.8 years	0.8 mg folic acid +0.5 mg vitamin B12 + 20 mg vitamin B6	2 years	Intervention group performed significantly well in memory tasks
Krikorian et al. [75]	Randomized placebo-controlled double blind trial	Diagnosis-MCI, n = 12 (intervention = 5, control = 7), mean age = 72.8 years	6–9 ml/kg of concord grape juice	12 weeks	Intervention group performed significantly well in memory tasks
Bo et al. [76]	Double blind randomized placebo-controlled trial	Diagnosis-MCI, n = 86 (intervention = 44, placebo = 42), mean age = 71 years	625 mg DHA + 600 mg EPA twice daily	6 months	Intervention group performed better in perceptual speed, visual memory, and working memory tasks
DeKosky et al. [77]	Double blind randomized placebo-controlled trial	Diagnosis-MCI, n = 482 (intervention = 256, control = 226) mean age = 79.1 years	120 mg of Gingko biloba extract twice daily	6.1 years	No significant effect in either the incidence of dementia or AD incidence
Peterson et al. [78]	Double blind randomized placebo-controlled trial	n = 769 (intervention = 257, donepezil group = 253, placebo = 259), mean age = 72.9 years	2000 IU of vitamin E daily v/s donepezil v/s placebo	3 years	There were no significant differences in the rate of progression to Alzheimer's disease between the vitamin E and placebo groups at any point.
Desideri et al. [79]	Double blind randomized parallel arm study	Diagnosis- MCI n = 90 (high v/s intermediate v/s low- 30 each) mean age = 71.2 years	Flavanol dose: High (990 mg/day) v/s intermediate (520 mg/day) v/s low (45 mg/day)	8 weeks	High dose flavanol group performed significantly well in executive function, processing speed, and verbal fluency
Ringman et al. [80]	Double blind randomized placebo-controlled study	Diagnosis- AD n = 36 mean age = 73.5 years	Curcumin dose 2–4 gram/day	24 weeks	Curcumin was generally well tolerated, but no significant benefits in AD in various cognitive tasks
Shults CW et al. [81]	Observational study	Diagnosis- Parkinson's disease (PD)	—	—	Levels of coenzyme Q10 in mitochondria was significantly lower in PD patients than controls
Evans et al. [82]	Randomized placebo-controlled trail	Study group- post menopausal women n = 80	Trans-resveratrol 150 mg/day	14 weeks	Resveratrol group did significantly better in cognitive tests such as verbal memory and overall cognitive performance

Study	Study type	Sample characteristics	Intervention	Study duration	Results
Tomata et al. [83]	Prospective cohort study	n = 13,988	3 arms: green tea consumption 1–2 cups /day v/s 3–4 cups/day v/s 5 or more cups/day	3 years	Green tea consumption is significantly associated with a lower risk of incident functional disability, even after adjustment for possible confounding factors.

Table 2.
An overview of few trials of nutraceuticals on various neurocognitive disorders, MCI, and healthy aging.

representative samples for better quality of results and translation into routine clinical practice [73]. The lack of adequate blinding, placebo response, mixed population, and clinical pragmatism limit the interpretation of these results. Hence, it is difficult to draw clinical implications. The overview of some of the studies has been depicted in **Table 2**.

4. Clinical utilities and advantages of nutraceuticals

Recently, there have been various small- and medium-size studies looking into the efficacy of nutraceuticals in the promotion of healthy aging, prevention of dementia in MCI subjects, and slowing down the progression of cognitive deficits in various neurocognitive disorders. In comparison with the pharmacological drugs that are being used for dementia, nutraceuticals bear many advantages:

- They are naturally occurring substances and are easily available in varieties of dietary constituents and formulae [84].
- The manufactured nutraceuticals may be easily available and procured from provisional stores or pharmacy counters as over-the-counter medications [85].
- Most of the nutraceuticals are taken orally, are easy to use, and are generally more acceptable.
- The preliminary trials have shown that these agents are safer to use in humans and will not cause any significant adverse effects [15, 17].
- In the current times of apparent therapeutic nihilism in the health professionals with regard to the pharmacological treatment options for neurocognitive disorders owing to the stagnation of new drug development, nutraceuticals may come handy in this respect [20].
- There is substantial scientific evidence on the mechanism of action of nutraceuticals through the studies in animal models [39, 62].
- The studies on pharmacodynamics and pharmacokinetic aspects of nutraceuticals in human subjects are going on.

- Any given nutraceutical may have multiple health benefits, such as the prevention and treatment of many chronic diseases such as diabetes, hypertension, heart diseases, atherosclerosis, musculoskeletal diseases, cancers, etc., along with neurocognitive disorders [85].

- Along with treatment aspects, nutraceuticals have a beneficial role in general health and well-being, healthy aging, and prevention and slowing down frailty in the elderly.

- Nutraceuticals may be well accepted by the general population and patients as they are naturally occurring, culturally ingrained in the given society, and devoid of the stigma associated with taking "artificial" medications.

5. Challenges and controversies of using nutraceuticals in clinical practice of dementia and healthy aging

The use of nutraceuticals is not free from challenges. These range from the point of production to the point of consumption and its effects on the human body as well as lack of a sound evidence base. Especially, when it comes to the aging spectrum, it is challenging to set arbitrary standpoints to assess cognitive status and effects of nutraceuticals. Another age-old challenge is the lack of standardized socioculturally sensitive cognitive assessment tools. Nutraceuticals are widely available in food products and often used over-the-counter; hence, the dose–response relationship is often obscure. Various caveats while discussing the role of nutraceuticals in healthy aging and neurocognitive disorders are the following:

- The results of interventional studies on the nutraceutical on various neurocognitive disorders are mixed across the board, and there is no emphatic evidence to support the use of nutraceuticals in these disorders [20].

- These studies have shown a marked placebo effect while treating patients with dementia and also in healthy aging [86].

- The ideal approach would be combining the nutrients together to match the physiological requirement of the body, which may be challenging, and manufacturing the complex mixture of various nutraceutical formulations may be cumbersome and costly [87]. It also makes it difficult to assess the efficacy of each constituent.

- There are challenges in analyzing the large data pertaining to the proportion of compositions of nutraceutical constituents in the food and assessing their qualities [88].

- The available questionnaires and rating scales on diet and nutritional intake for monitoring of the effects of nutraceuticals are prone to recall bias and may have confounding effects on the study results [20].

- Testing the baseline nutrient levels of the nutraceuticals in the body and personalized medicine and a more targeted approach by prescribing the nutraceuticals based on specific nutritional deficiencies is required in the current scenario of precision medicine practice [87].

- The setting of an appropriate dosing regimen may be difficult due to erratic patterns of metabolism, poor blood–brain barrier penetration, nonspecific targeting, and reduced bioavailability.

- Neurocognitive disorders are common in older people. Old age is associated with changes in pharmacodynamics and pharmacodynamics that can influence the bioavailability, metabolism, and, eventually, the action of all drugs. Adverse effects of medicines and toxicity are, hence, more frequent [2, 3, 7]. In addition, the central nervous system is more vulnerable to the effects of any drug in dementia, and dosing needs supervision as functional capacity declines gradually with dementia progression. Without standard guidelines, it becomes difficult to decide appropriate dosing regimen for nutraceuticals in older people (especially in those living with dementia), which is safe and well tolerated [84, 85]. More research is warranted to understand the safety of ingestion of nutraceutical-based products in old age. Another related concern is drug–drug interactions as polypharmacy is a rule rather than exception in later life.

- There is a lack of standardized treatment guidelines for the use of nutraceuticals [21, 56]. This leads to wide variation and subjectivity in their dosing and usage.

- Further studies are required to look into the pharmacokinetic and pharmacodynamic profile of nutraceuticals specifically in humans [21].

- There is a need for robust evidence for the regulated regimens of nutraceutical prescription including dose, duration, and knowledge of adverse reactions with post-marketing surveillance.

- The nutrient mixtures are not free from various contaminants, such as allergens, natural and unintended contaminants, heavy metals, pesticides and herbicides, mycotoxins, natural plant toxins, microbiological agents, marine toxins, etc., which can be harmful to humans and need to be purified before marketing [85].

- The potential interactions of nutraceuticals with other drugs and supplements need to be studied.

- The long-term impact of continued nutraceutical intake needs to be studied [84].

- As most of the nutraceuticals are available as over-the-counter supplements, there is a risk of abuse and toxicity [63].

- Inertia among clinicians regarding their use, misinterpretation of their role as "placebo," which is further perpetuated by the lack of strong evidence base.

- There are multiple other factors that can influence aging and the trajectory of neurocognitive disorders (such as age, gender, substance use, education status, cognitive and leisure-time activities, exercise, diet patterns, social connectivity, sleep, relationships, and stress levels). Many trials involving nutraceuticals either do not take these factors into account or are too stringent about inclusion criteria, which makes the study population nonrepresentative of clinical settings [73, 87]. This makes the findings difficult to interpret. The complex interplay between all these modifiable and nonmodifiable factors in aging can potentially modify the influence of nutraceuticals, which needs further research.

- There is a need for the development, implementation, and evaluation of public health strategies for improving nutrition in the general population [21].

6. Conclusion and future direction

Nutraceuticals are naturally derived bioactive compounds that are found in foods, dietary supplements, and herbal products and have health promoting, disease preventing, or medicinal properties. They have multiple actions, including anti-inflammatory, antioxidant, anticarcinogenic, and antimicrobial properties. The field of nutraceutical psychiatry is relatively new and is slowly seeping into the mainstream psychiatric practice because of a number of recent studies that have established some efficacy in the prevention and treatment of neurocognitive disorders, slowing the progression of MCI into dementia and promotion of healthy aging. However, these studies are significantly heterogeneous in terms of methodology, sample selection, assessment, and dose and formulations of nutraceuticals with largely mixed results. We are lacking robust scientific evidence for the efficacy of nutraceuticals in cognitive neurology and psychiatry. Till date, nutraceuticals continue to be used as adjuvants or over-the-counter products for healthy aging as well as the prevention and management of dementia.

We need more large-sized randomized controlled trials for the better establishment of the efficacy of the nutraceuticals in neurocognitive disorders. The molecular basis of the action of nutraceuticals in human subjects needs to be unraveled for a better understanding of these molecules. The composition of each supplement must be carefully studied, and there has to be a rigorous regulatory mechanism for dosing, purification, mixing the different compounds, manufacturing, prescription, and marketing of these compounds that are backed by scientific evidence. Further studies are required for personalized medicine based on the physiological requirement of the body after testing for the blood levels of the nutraceuticals. From a public health perspective, the public and the health professionals need to be educated regarding the healthy nutrition and the availability of various nutraceuticals, and the policies pertaining to the regulation of sales of these compounds need to be formulated. Notwithstanding all limitations, nutraceuticals hold an immense promise in the field of healthy aging and disorders related to age. A deeper understanding of the nuances related to the mechanism of action, dosage, composition, role in different time periods of life, and, finally, other physiological effects will improvise their role in preventive and aging medicine. Age-appropriate guidelines can then be put into practice to help clinicians worldwide with their use. Whether nutraceuticals work in neurodegenerative conditions, especially dementia, stands the test of time, but based on the available evidence, it is definitely worth a try!

Author contributions

Both the authors have contributed equally to the conceptualization, design, literature review, drafting and editing the manuscript. The final version has been agreed upon by both the authors.

Conflict of interest

None.

Funding

None to disclose.

Author details

Abhishek Ramesh[1] and Debanjan Banerjee[2]*

1 Department of Psychiatry, Adichunchanagiri Institute of Medical Sciences, Mandya, Karnataka, India

2 Consultant Geriatric Psychiatrist, ASHA THE HOPE, Kolkata, India

*Address all correspondence to: dr.djan88@gmail.com

References

[1] Gilbert SF. Aging: The Biology of Senescence. Dev Biol 6th Ed [Internet]. 2000 [cited 2022 Feb 27]; Available from: https://www.ncbi.nlm.nih.gov/books/NBK10041/

[2] Fontana L. Modulating human aging and age-associated diseases. Biochimica et Biophysica Acta. 2009;**1790**(10):1133-1138

[3] da Costa JP, Vitorino R, Silva GM, Vogel C, Duarte AC, Rocha-Santos T. A synopsis on aging—Theories, mechanisms and future prospects. Ageing Research Reviews. 2016;**29**:90-112

[4] Baltes BB, Rudolph CW, Bal AC. A review of aging theories and modern work perspectives. In: The Oxford Handbook of Work and Aging. New York, NY, US: Oxford University Press; 2012. pp. 117-136. (Oxford library of psychology)

[5] Luo J, Mills K, le Cessie S, Noordam R, van Heemst D. Ageing, age-related diseases and oxidative stress: What to do next? Ageing Research Reviews. 2020;**57**:100982

[6] Edes AN, Crews DE. Allostatic load and biological anthropology. American Journal of Physical Anthropology. 2017;**162**(Suppl. 63):44-70

[7] Slagboom PE, Vijg J. Genetic instability and aging: Theories, facts, and future perspectives. Genome. 1989;**31**(1):373-385

[8] Shay JW. Telomeres and aging. Current Opinion in Cell Biology. 2018;**52**:1-7

[9] Reynolds JC, Bwiza CP, Lee C. Mitonuclear genomics and aging. Human Genetics. 2020;**139**(3):381-399

[10] Wang X, Ma Z, Cheng J, Lv Z. A genetic program theory of aging using an RNA population model. Ageing Research Reviews. 2014;**13**:46-54

[11] Tucker-Drob EM. Cognitive aging and dementia: A life span perspective. Annu Rev Dev Psychol. 2019;**1**:177-196

[12] Baghel MS, Singh P, Srivas S, Thakur MK. Cognitive changes with aging. Proc Natl Acad Sci India Sect B Biol Sci. 2019;**89**(3):765-773

[13] Singh P, Sivanandam TM, Konar A, Thakur MK. Role of nutraceuticals in cognition during aging and related disorders. Neurochemistry International. 2021;**143**:104928

[14] Tucker KL. Nutrient intake, nutritional status, and cognitive function with aging. Annals of the New York Academy of Sciences. 2016;**1367**(1):38-49

[15] Mondello L. Nutraceuticals and separations. Analytical and Bioanalytical Chemistry. 2013;**405**(13):4589-4590

[16] Kalra EK. Nutraceutical--definition and introduction. AAPS PharmSci. 2003;**5**(3):E25

[17] Siddiqui RA, Moghadasian MH. Nutraceuticals and nutrition supplements: Challenges and opportunities. Nutrients. 2020;**12**(6):1593

[18] Dickinson A, Blatman J, El-Dash N, Franco JC. Consumer usage and reasons for using dietary supplements: Report of a series of surveys. Journal of the American College of Nutrition. 2014;**33**(2):176-182

[19] Nicoletti M. Nutraceuticals and botanicals: Overview and perspectives.

International Journal of Food Sciences and Nutrition. 2012;**63**(Suppl. 1):2-6

[20] Sarris J. Nutritional psychiatry: From concept to the clinic. Drugs. 2019;**79**(9):929-934

[21] Jacka FN. Nutritional psychiatry: Where to next? eBioMedicine. 2017;**17**:24-29

[22] Lakhan SE, Vieira KF. Nutritional therapies for mental disorders. Nutrition Journal. 2008;**21**(7):2

[23] Dhan Prakash DP, Charu Gupta CG. Role of antioxidant polyphenols in nutraceuticals and human health. In: Prakash D, Sharma G, editors. Phytochemicals of Nutraceutical Importance [Internet]. Wallingford: CABI; 2014 [cited 2022 Feb 27]. pp. 208-228. Available from: http://www.cabi.org/cabebooks/ebook/20143083518

[24] Scalbert A, Manach C, Morand C, Rémésy C, Jiménez L. Dietary polyphenols and the prevention of diseases. Critical Reviews in Food Science and Nutrition. 2005;**45**(4):287-306

[25] Dhan Prakash DP, Charu Gupta CG. Carotenoids: Chemistry and health benefits. In: Prakash D, Sharma G, editors. Phytochemicals of Nutraceutical Importance [Internet]. Wallingford: CABI; 2014 [cited 2022 Feb 27]. pp. 181-195. Available from: http://www.cabi.org/cabebooks/ebook/20143083516

[26] Masson L. Phytosterols and their healthy effects. In: Prakash D, Sharma G, editors. Phytochemicals of Nutraceutical Importance [Internet]. Wallingford: CABI; 2014 [cited 2022 Feb 27]. pp. 173-80. Available from: http://www.cabi.org/cabebooks/ebook/20143083515

[27] Singh RL, Vishwakarma SP, Pankaj Singh PS. Vitamins and minerals: roles and plant sources. In: Prakash D, Sharma G, editors. Phytochemicals of nutraceutical importance [Internet]. Wallingford: CABI; 2014 [cited 2022 Feb 27]. pp. 310-23. Available from: http://www.cabi.org/cabebooks/ebook/20143083523

[28] Gupta C, Prakash D. Nutraceuticals for geriatrics. Journal of Traditional and Complementary Medicine. 2015;**5**(1):5-14

[29] Masson L. Omega 3 and omega 6 fatty acids in human health. In: Prakash D, Sharma G, editors. Phytochemicals of Nutraceutical Importance [Internet]. Wallingford: CABI; 2014 [cited 2022 Feb 27]. pp. 116-31. Available from: http://www.cabi.org/cabebooks/ebook/20143083512

[30] Charu Gupta CG, Dhan Prakash DP, Rostagno MH, Callaway TR. Synbiotics: promoting gastrointestinal health. In: Prakash D, Sharma G, editors. Phytochemicals of Nutraceutical Importance [Internet]. Wallingford: CABI; 2014 [cited 2022 Feb 27]. pp. 61-78. Available from: http://www.cabi.org/cabebooks/ebook/20143083509

[31] Prasad AS. Zinc: Role in immunity, oxidative stress and chronic inflammation. Current Opinion in Clinical Nutrition and Metabolic Care. 2009;**12**(6):646-652

[32] Wu T-Y, Chen C-P, Jinn T-R. Traditional Chinese medicines and Alzheimer's disease. Taiwanese Journal of Obstetrics & Gynecology. 2011;**50**(2):131-135

[33] He X, Liu RH. Cranberry phytochemicals: Isolation, structure elucidation, and their antiproliferative and antioxidant activities. Journal of Agricultural and Food Chemistry. 2006;**54**(19):7069-7074

[34] Boots AW, Haenen GRMM, Bast A. Health effects of quercetin: From antioxidant to nutraceutical. European Journal of Pharmacology. 2008;**585**(2-3):325-337

[35] Chiu H-F, Venkatakrishnan K, Wang C-K. The role of nutraceuticals as a complementary therapy against various neurodegenerative diseases: A mini-review. Journal of Traditional and Complementary Medicine. 2020;**10**(5):434-439

[36] Canevelli M, Lucchini F, Quarata F, Bruno G, Cesari M. Nutrition and dementia: Evidence for preventive approaches? Nutrients. 2016;**8**(3):144

[37] Vranesić-Bender D. The role of nutraceuticals in anti-aging medicine. Acta Clinica Croatica. 2010;**49**(4):537-544

[38] Bhat RS, Chiu E, Jeste DV. Nutrition and geriatric psychiatry: A neglected field. Current Opinion in Psychiatry. 2005;**18**(6):609-614

[39] Makkar R, Behl T, Bungau S, Zengin G, Mehta V, Kumar A, et al. Nutraceuticals in neurological disorders. International Journal of Molecular Sciences. 2020;**21**(12):E4424

[40] Dutta S, Roy S, Roy S. Functional foods for mental health promotion. J Mahatma Gandhi Inst Med Sci. 2020;**25**(2):72

[41] Farooqui AA, Farooqui T, Madan A, Ong JH-J, Ong W-Y. Ayurvedic medicine for the treatment of dementia: Mechanistic aspects. Evid-Based Complement Altern Med ECAM. 2018;**2018**:2481076

[42] Das L, Bhaumik E, Raychaudhuri U, Chakraborty R. Role of nutraceuticals in human health. Journal of Food Science and Technology. 2012;**49**(2):173-183

[43] Dkhar P, Sharma R. Beneficial effects of nutraceuticals in healthy brain aging. In: Nutraceuticals in Brain Health and Beyond [Internet]. Elsevier; 2021 [cited 2022 Mar 3]. pp. 125-39. Available from: https://linkinghub.elsevier.com/retrieve/pii/B9780128205938000094

[44] Haldar S, Ghosh S, Kumar V, Saini S, Lahiri D, Roy P. Chapter 29 - Nutraceuticals in brain health. In: Ghosh D, editor. Nutraceuticals in Brain Health and Beyond [Internet]. Academic Press; 2021 [cited 2022 May 9]. p. 409-39. Available from: https://www.sciencedirect.com/science/article/pii/B978012820593800029X

[45] Hodjat M, Khalid M, Asghari M, Atri S, Rahimifard M, Nejad SM, et al. Nutrients and Nutraceuticals in Aging. In: Nabavi SM, D'Onofrio G, Nabavi SF, editors. Nutrients and Nutraceuticals for Active & Healthy Ageing [Internet]. Singapore: Springer; 2020 [cited 2022 May 9]. p. 63-109. Available from: https://doi.org/10.1007/978-981-15-3552-9_5

[46] Bayrami Z, Khalid M, Asgari Dastjerdi S, Sadat Masjedi M. Functional Foods and Dietary Patterns for Prevention of Cognitive Decline in Aging. In: Nabavi SM, D'Onofrio G, Nabavi SF, editors. Nutrients and Nutraceuticals for Active & Healthy Ageing [Internet]. Singapore: Springer; 2020 [cited 2022 May 9]. p. 217-238. Available from: https://doi.org/10.1007/978-981-15-3552-9_10

[47] Howes M-J, Perry N, Vásquez-Londoño C, Perry E. Role of phytochemicals as nutraceuticals for cognitive functions affected in ageing. British Journal of Pharmacology. 2019;**25**:177

[48] Hang L, Basil AH, Lim K-L. Nutraceuticals in Parkinson's disease. Neuromolecular Medicine. 2016;**18**(3):306-321

[49] Lama A, Pirozzi C, Avagliano C, Annunziata C, Mollica M, Calignano A, et al. Nutraceuticals: An integrative approach to starve Parkinson's disease. Brain Behav Immun - Health. 2020;**1**(2):100037

[50] Mythri RB, Joshi AK, Bharath MMS. Chapter 44 - Nutraceuticals and Other Natural Products in Parkinson's Disease Therapy: Focus on Clinical Applications. In: Watson RR, Preedy VR, editors. Bioactive Nutraceuticals and Dietary Supplements in Neurological and Brain Disease [Internet]. San Diego: Academic Press; 2015 [cited 2022 May 9]. p. 421-431. Available from: https://www.sciencedirect.com/science/article/pii/B9780124114623000448

[51] Alfieri A, Mann GE. Chapter 37 - Bioactive Nutraceuticals and Stroke: Activation of Endogenous Antioxidant Pathways and Molecular Mechanisms Underlying Neurovascular Protection. In: Watson RR, Preedy VR, editors. Bioactive Nutraceuticals and Dietary Supplements in Neurological and Brain Disease [Internet]. San Diego: Academic Press; 2015 [cited 2022 May 9]. p. 365-379. Available from: https://www.sciencedirect.com/science/article/pii/B9780124114623000370

[52] Chang D, Liu J, Bilinski K, Xu L, Steiner GZ, Seto SW, et al. Herbal medicine for the treatment of vascular dementia: An overview of scientific evidence. Evid-Based Complement Altern Med ECAM. 2016;**2016**:7293626

[53] Zhou X, Seto SW, Chang D, Kiat H, Razmovski-Naumovski V, Chan K, et al. Synergistic effects of Chinese herbal medicine: A comprehensive review of methodology and current research. Frontiers in Pharmacology. 2016;**12**(7):201

[54] Gu P, Chen H. Modern bioinformatics meets traditional Chinese medicine. Briefings in Bioinformatics. 2014;**15**(6):984-1003

[55] Small BJ, Rawson KS, Martin C, Eisel SL, Sanberg CD, McEvoy CL, et al. Nutraceutical intervention improves older adults' cognitive functioning. Rejuvenation Research. 2014;**17**(1):27-32

[56] Chelluboina B, Vemuganti R. Therapeutic potential of nutraceuticals to protect brain after stroke. Neurochemistry International. 2021;**142**:104908

[57] Yu M, Bega D. A review of the clinical evidence for complementary and alternative medicine in Huntington's disease. Tremor Hyperkinetic Mov N Y N. 2019:1-9

[58] Banerjee S, Dutta S, Ghosh S, Sil PC. Chapter 17 - Nutraceuticals in neurodegenerative diseases. In: Ghosh D, editor. Nutraceuticals in Brain Health and Beyond [Internet]. Academic Press; 2021 [cited 2022 May 9]. p. 249-70. Available from: https://www.sciencedirect.com/science/article/pii/B9780128205938000173

[59] Pardini M, Serrati C, Guida S, Mattei C, Abate L, Massucco D, et al. Souvenaid reduces behavioral deficits and improves social cognition skills in frontotemporal dementia: A proof-of-concept study. Neurodegenerative Diseases. 2015;**15**(1):58-62

[60] Peysselon F, Ricard-Blum S. Understanding the biology of aging with interaction networks. Maturitas. 2011;**69**(2):126-130

[61] Kenyon CJ. The genetics of ageing. Nature. 2010;**464**(7288):504-512

[62] Dong Y, Guha S, Sun X, Cao M, Wang X, Zou S. Nutraceutical interventions for promoting healthy aging in invertebrate models. Oxidative

Medicine and Cellular Longevity. 2012;**2012**(718491):1-10

[63] Chiappedi M, de Vincenzi S, Bejor M. Nutraceuticals in psychiatric practice. Recent Patents CNS Drug Discov. 2012;**7**(2):163-172

[64] Lucas G. Gut thinking: The gut microbiome and mental health beyond the head. Microbial Ecology in Health and Disease. 2018;**29**(2):1548250

[65] Bull MJ, Plummer NT. Part 1: The human gut microbiome in health and disease. Integr Med Clin J. 2014;**13**(6):17-22

[66] Cheung SG, Goldenthal AR, Uhlemann A-C, Mann JJ, Miller JM, Sublette ME. Systematic review of gut microbiota and major depression. Front Psychiatry [Internet]. 11 Feb 2019;**10**(34):1-17

[67] Penner R, Fedorak RN, Madsen KL. Probiotics and nutraceuticals: Non-medicinal treatments of gastrointestinal diseases. Current Opinion in Pharmacology. 2005;**5**(6):596-603

[68] Catinean A, Neag MA, Muntean DM, Bocsan IC, Buzoianu AD. An overview on the interplay between nutraceuticals and gut microbiota. PeerJ. 2018;**6**:e4465

[69] Carabotti M, Scirocco A, Maselli MA, Severi C. The gut-brain axis: Interactions between enteric microbiota, central and enteric nervous systems. Annals of Gastroenterology. 2015;**28**(2):203-209

[70] Laparra JM, Sanz Y. Interactions of gut microbiota with functional food components and nutraceuticals. Pharmacological Research. 2010;**61**(3): 219-225

[71] Lyte M. Microbial endocrinology: Host-microbiota neuroendocrine interactions influencing brain and behavior. Gut Microbes. 2014;**5**(3):381-389

[72] McGrattan AM, McEvoy CT, McGuinness B, McKinley MC, Woodside JV. Effect of dietary interventions in mild cognitive impairment: A systematic review. The British Journal of Nutrition. 2018;**120**(12):1388-1405

[73] Mecocci P, Tinarelli C, Schulz RJ, Polidori MC. Nutraceuticals in cognitive impairment and Alzheimer's disease. Frontiers in Pharmacology. 2014;**5**:147

[74] de Jager CA, Oulhaj A, Jacoby R, Refsum H, Smith AD. Cognitive and clinical outcomes of homocysteine-lowering B-vitamin treatment in mild cognitive impairment: A randomized controlled trial. International Journal of Geriatric Psychiatry. 2012;**27**(6):592-600

[75] Krikorian R, Nash TA, Shidler MD, Shukitt-Hale B, Joseph JA. Concord grape juice supplementation improves memory function in older adults with mild cognitive impairment. The British Journal of Nutrition. 2010;**103**(5):730-734

[76] Bo Y, Zhang X, Wang Y, You J, Cui H, Zhu Y, et al. The n-3 polyunsaturated fatty acids supplementation improved the cognitive function in the Chinese elderly with mild cognitive impairment: A double-blind randomized controlled trial. Nutrients. 2017;**9**(1):E54

[77] DeKosky ST, Williamson JD, Fitzpatrick AL, Kronmal RA, Ives DG, Saxton JA, et al. Ginkgo biloba for prevention of dementia: A randomized controlled trial. JAMA. 2008;**300**(19): 2253-2262

[78] Petersen RC, Thomas RG, Grundman M, Bennett D, Doody R, Ferris S, et al. Vitamin E and donepezil for the treatment of mild cognitive

impairment. The New England Journal of Medicine. 2005;**352**(23):2379-2388

[79] Desideri G, Kwik-Uribe C, Grassi D, Necozione S, Ghiadoni L, Mastroiacovo D, et al. Benefits in cognitive function, blood pressure, and insulin resistance through cocoa flavanol consumption in elderly subjects with mild cognitive impairment: The cocoa, cognition, and aging (CoCoA) study. Hypertens Dallas Tex 1979. 2012;**60**(3):794-801

[80] Ringman JM, Frautschy SA, Teng E, Begum AN, Bardens J, Beigi M, et al. Oral curcumin for Alzheimer's disease: Tolerability and efficacy in a 24-week randomized, double blind, placebo-controlled study. Alzheimer's Research & Therapy. 2012;**4**(5):43

[81] Shults CW, Haas RH, Passov D, Beal MF. Coenzyme Q10 levels correlate with the activities of complexes I and II/III in mitochondria from parkinsonian and nonparkinsonian subjects. Annals of Neurology. 1997;**42**(2):261-264

[82] Evans HM, Howe PRC, Wong RHX. Effects of resveratrol on cognitive performance, mood and cerebrovascular function in post-menopausal women; A 14-week randomised placebo-controlled intervention trial. Nutrients. 2017;**9**(1):E27

[83] Tomata Y, Kakizaki M, Nakaya N, Tsuboya T, Sone T, Kuriyama S, et al. Green tea consumption and the risk of incident functional disability in elderly Japanese: The Ohsaki cohort 2006 study. The American Journal of Clinical Nutrition. 2012;**95**(3):732-739

[84] Helal NA, Eassa HA, Amer AM, Eltokhy MA, Edafiogho I, Nounou MI. Nutraceuticals' novel formulations: The good, the bad, the unknown and patents involved. Recent Patents on Drug Delivery & Formulation. 2019;**13**(2):105-156

[85] Bagchi D, Preuss HG, Swaroop A, editors. Nutraceuticals and Functional Foods in Human Health and Disease Prevention. 1st ed. CRC Press. 2015. DOI: 10.1201/b19308

[86] Weimer K, Colloca L, Enck P. Placebo effects in psychiatry: Mediators and moderators. Lancet Psychiatry. 2015;**2**(3):246-257

[87] Sarris J, Logan AC, Akbaraly TN, Amminger GP, Balanzá-Martínez V, Freeman MP, et al. Nutritional medicine as mainstream in psychiatry. Lancet Psychiatry. 2015;**2**(3):271-274

[88] Quirk SE, Williams LJ, O'Neil A, Pasco JA, Jacka FN, Housden S, et al. The association between diet quality, dietary patterns and depression in adults: A systematic review. BMC Psychiatry. 2013;**27**(13):175

Section 4

Assisted Living: Technology for Healthy Aging

Chapter 8

Perspective Chapter: Telehealth Technologies for the Elderly People

Ahmadreza Shamsabadi, Esmaeil Mehraeen and Zahra Pashaei

Abstract

Home telehealth technology delivers a telemedicine tool for elder adults to take an active role in the management of their chronic diseases. This study aimed to determine the requirements and applications of home telehealth systems to monitor health parameters of the elderly. Electronic databases including PubMed, Scopus, Web of Science complemented by Google Scholar were searched. This systematic review was conducted based on preferred reporting items for systematic reviews and meta-analyses. In this study, 21 articles met the inclusion criteria and were included in the final review. There were 80 different requirements and 15 types of applications to create a home telehealth system specifically for the elderly. The highest frequency of applications element was related to the "blood pressure" (18%) and the lowest frequency related to items such as blood coagulation (1%) monitoring. Other systems` elements were "alert system" (12%), "information analysis" (12%), smartphone (20%), and internet (23%). Recognizing all used requirements and achieved capabilities may assist in designing more effective systems. They might be expanded at national level to meet the elderly's needs at a greater scale.

Keywords: elderly, home care service, nursing informatics, telehealth, system requirement

1. Introduction

The population of elderly is increasingly rising [1, 2]. In 2011, there were about 657 million elderly people in the world, and in 2050, their population is expected to reach about 1.91 billion [3]. Elder adult patients are more affected by multiple acute and chronic conditions and diseases requiring continuous care. This management might be provided by a variety of medical and health professionals in different settings [4, 5]. Over the past few decades, there has been a widespread prevalence of chronic diseases including diabetes, chronic obstructive pulmonary disease (COPD), and cardiovascular diseases in elderly, due to increased life period [6]. Among elderly, chronic diseases that occur simultaneously have increased and caused limitation in their physical activities, social interactions, and general health [7]. This will increase the need of long-term care for elderly [8].

Telehealth (also known as remote health) has been defined as intermediations that allow send and receive remote of health data and supplementary information between a patient and healthcare expert(s) to support in the diagnosis and managing of health situation [9]. Telehealth in general refers to several technologies, systems, and applications that could be adopted to provide remote support of health care at home [10]. This requires a set of fundamental functionalities, such as remote consultation and diagnosis, as well as the possibility of data gathering for the monitoring of health dimensions and vital signs (e.g., blood pressure, heart rate, and seizure risk). Home telehealth (HTH) is described as "the use of telecommunications by a home care provider to link patients or customers to one or more out-of-home sources of care information, education, or service by means of telephones, computers, interactive television, or some combination of each" [11].

There are several telehealth service delivery models, and each model has different requirements and attributes [12]. Various review studies address information and communication technology (ICT) applications to support elder adult's telehealth at home. The main focuses of these studies include patient self-management [13], ethical considerations [14], facilitators and barriers to telehealth applications [15], elder adult's points of view about ICT applications [16], digital technology for aging in place [17], general review of monitoring technologies [18], and telephone application for communication between nurses and elderly [19]. Therefore, it turns out that there is a lack of review studies in the area of home telehealth system requirements for elderly. This study intends to focus systematically on evidences and experiences to determine applications and requirements of home telehealth system for elderly.

2. Methods

2.1 Aims

This study was to determine the requirements and applications of home telehealth systems to design and development of an effective system for telemonitoring of health parameters for elderly living at home.

2.2 Design

A systematic literature review of evidence and experiences.

2.3 Search methods

An electronic search was carried out in four scientific databases including Scopus, Web of Science and PubMed, Google scholar for English language studies. A researcher with a health information management degree (ARS) designed a Boolean search strategy. Compositions of the following search terms were used:

a. elderly OR frail elderly OR old adult OR geriatric OR aged

b. health information management OR remainder system OR wireless devise OR sensors

c. telemonitoring OR telemedicine OR home care OR home nursing OR home telehealth

d. (a) AND (b) AND (c)

2.4 Inclusion criteria

The inclusion criteria were original articles describing telehealth systems for monitoring elderly's health at home published in English language. Only articles that applied a remote monitoring system for elderly living at home were selected and analyzed.

2.5 Exclusion criteria

Exclusion criteria were studies published in a language other than English, studies published before 2013, studies with no full-text available, and any type of publication other than original article including review papers, conference abstracts, letters, etc. Papers that focused only on those systems aimed to monitor the environmental factors of elderly for remote home monitoring purposes were also excluded.

2.6 Search outcomes

In total, 1727 records were retrieved by searching the formerly mentioned databases. From articles found, first, duplicates were removed. Then, the titles and abstracts were screened by two researchers (SRNK, ARS) conforming to the inclusion/exclusion criteria. In this study, 21 articles met the inclusion criteria and were included in the final review. The process of PRISMA[1] for data collection and analysis was applied (**Figure 1**).

2.7 Quality appraisal

The full texts of potentially related article were separately evaluated by the same two researchers independently. Contradictions were solved in consultation with researchers who also examined and authenticated the relatedness of all included articles.

2.8 Data abstraction

Data elements were extracted from selected articles. The extracted criteria were then reviewed by an expert panel including two medical informatics specialists and three health information management specialists who have been involved with other elderly informatics projects. The final classification obtained based on the five researchers' agreement is presented in **Table 1**.

2.9 Synthesis

The selected articles were analyzed based on five main data variables presenting the applications and requirements of home telehealth monitoring systems for elderly including: applications, nonfunctional requirements (system-oriented and technical features), functional requirements (user-oriented features), devices, and communication infrastructures obtained from telehealth service delivery models and system requirements engineering [40].

---

[1] Preferred reporting items for systematic reviews and meta-analyses.

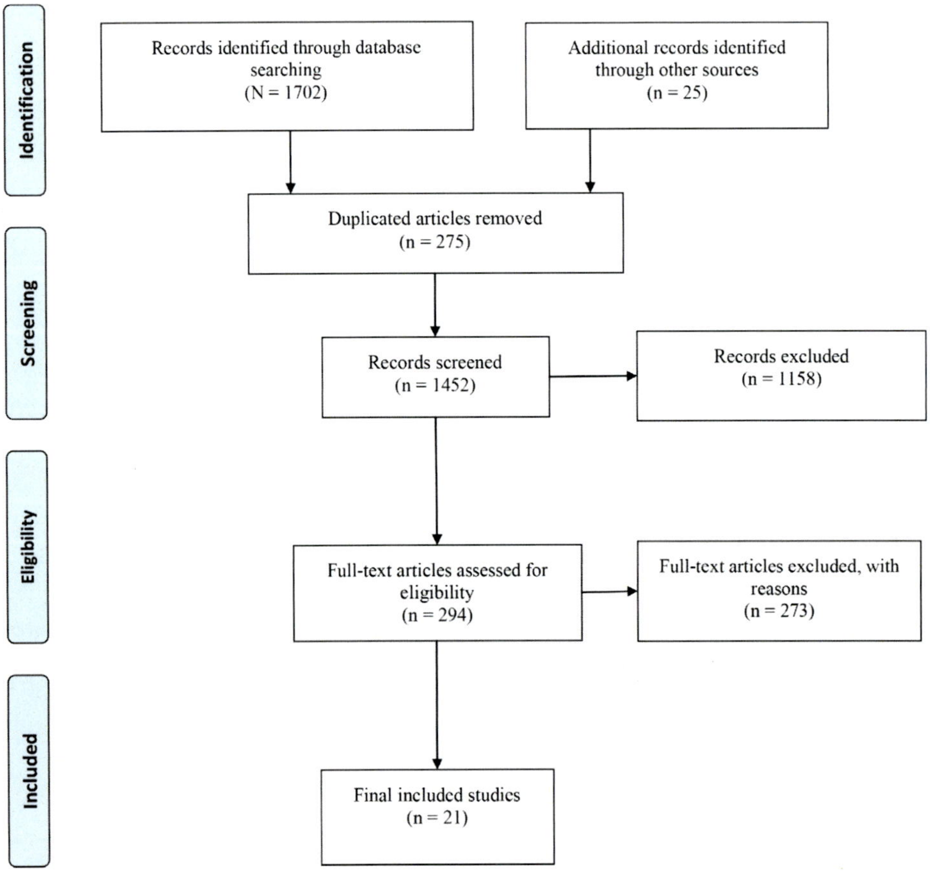

Figure 1.
The process of PRISMA for data collection and analysis.

3. Results

Table 1 presents the specific extracted data from the given papers based on seven data element of date of publication, country or project name, applications, nonfunctional requirement, functional requirement, device, and communication infrastructure.

In this study, five different aspects of home telehealth systems designed for aged monitoring were considered and analyzed. These aspects include (a) applications: indicating the purpose of using the system; (b) functional requirement: defines system performance and describes the inputs, behaviors, and outputs of the system for the user [41]; (c) nonfunctional requirement: refers to system architecture made of technical and operational features to make functional requirement working properly [42]; (d) device: specifying the tools that have been mostly used in the systems; and (e) communication infrastructure: implying to the type of networks and the way the information is mostly transmitted from the elderly's home to the central system and roaming from this station to the other parts of the system. Here, we give more information about each of aspects used for mentioned home telehealth system in detail.

According to the data analysis, it was revealed that the most common applications of home telehealth systems were respectively blood pressure (18%) and heart rate

First author (Reference)	Country/Project	Applications (Usages)	Nonfunctional requirements	Functional requirements	Devices	Communication infrastructures
Madigan E [20]	Ohio/ Telecare	1. Blood pressure M*[1] 2. Heart rate M 3. Weight M 4. Oxygen saturation M	1. Central database 2. Guideline and standard observation	1. Education for the users	1. Land line phone	1. Phone line
Rantz MJ [21]	Missouri	1. Blood pressure M 2. Oxygen saturation M 3. Blood sugar M 4. Respiration M 5. Restlessness M	1. Central database 2. Guideline and standard observation 3. Information analysis 4. User-friendliness 5. EPR and PHR development 6. Applying e-mail 7. Web-based design 8. Management of apps 9. Intelligent performance 10. System security	1. Detection of emergency situation 2. Reminder system 3. Alert system 4. Display information for the users 5. Ubiquitous information access	1. Bio-medical sensors 2. Plus-Doppler radar 3. Camera	1. Internet
Katalinic O [22]	Australia	1. Blood pressure M 2. Weight M 3. Oxygen saturation M 4. Heart rate M	1. Guideline and standard observation 2. Information analysis 3. User-friendliness 4. Applying e-mail 5. Applying videoconference 6. Applying web portal 7. Management of apps 8. System security	1. Education for the users 2. Social and emotional support 3. Personalized services	1. Intel health guide[2] 2. Apple iPod 3. Broad band router 4. Smart phone 5. PC 6. Web-cam 7. e-book reader	1. Internet
Dhillon JS [23]	Malaysia	1. Blood pressure M 2. Weight M 3. Physical activity M 4. Diet tracking M	1. Central database 2. Information analysis 3. User-friendliness 4. Applying e-mail 5. Web-based design 6. Applying videoconference	1. Education for the users 2. Reminder system 3. Alert system 4. Display information for the users 5. Ubiquitous information access	1. Apple iPod 2. Web-cam 3. Smart phone 4. PC 5. Game controllers	1. Internet

First author (Reference)	Country/Project	Applications (Usages)	Nonfunctional requirements	Functional requirements	Devices	Communication infrastructures
			7. Applying web portal 8. Applying video linked 9. Applying virtual environment 10. Management of apps 11. Open and extensible development 12. Real-time monitoring 13. Intelligent performance 14. System security 15. Make social connection	6. Social and emotional support 7. Motivation creation 8. Personalized services 9. Playing remotely game 10. Creation user profile		
Vaidehi V [24]	India	1. Blood pressure M 2. Heart rate M 3. Respiration M 4. Body temperature M	1. Central database 2. Information analysis 3. User-friendliness 4. Data reduction ability 5. Agent-based design 6. Intelligent performance 7. System security	1. Display information for the users	1. Bio-medical sensors	1. Internet 2. Wi-Fi &Wi-Max
Lamprinakos G [25]	Athens Greece/ inCASA	1. Blood pressure M 2. Weight M 3. Oxygen saturation M 4. Blood sugar M 5. Heart rate M 6. Physical activity M 7. Blood coagulation M	1. Central database 2. Information analysis 3. User-friendliness 4. EPR and PHR development 5. Web-based design 6. Guideline and standard observation 7. Applying web portal 8. Applying audio message 9. Applying POP – UP[3] 10. Management of apps 11. UPnP technology[4] based design 12. Real-time monitoring	1. Education for the users 2. Detection of emergency situation 3. Reminder system 4. Alert system 5. Display information for the users 6. Ubiquitous information access 7. Personalized services 8. Creation user profile 9. Social & emotional support	1. Bio-medical sensors 2. Smart phone 3. PC 4. Activity hub 5. IoT device	1. Internet 2. Wi-Fi &Wi-Max 3. SMS 4. Bluetooth

First author (Reference)	Country/Project	Applications (Usages)	Nonfunctional requirements	Functional requirements	Devices	Communication infrastructures
			13. Intelligent performance 14. Service-oriented 15. System security			
Chung Y-F [26]	Taiwan	1. Blood pressure M 2. Respiration M 3. Heart rate M 4. Oxygen saturation M 5. Physical activity M 6. Body temperature M 7. ECG M	1. Central database 2. Information analysis 3. EPR and PHR development 4. Applying e-mail 5. Web-based design 6. Applying video linked 7. Management of apps 8. Real-time monitoring 9. Intelligent performance 10. System security	1. Education for the users 2. Detection of emergency situation 3. Reminder system 4. Alert system 5. Display information for the users 6. Ubiquitous information access 7. Graphical representation of outputs	1. Bio-medical sensors 2. Smart phone 3. PC 4. Camera 5. RFID reader	1. Internet 2. Wi-Fi &Wi-Max 3. SMS 4. Bluetooth 5. RFID[5] 6. 6- Zig bee[6]
Tseng KC [27]	China	1. Blood pressure M 2. Physical activity M	1. Central database 2. Information analysis 3. User friendliness 4. EPR and PHR development 5. Web-based design 6. Applying audio message 7. Applying animated graphics 8. Management of apps 9. Real-time monitoring 10. Intelligent performance 11. System security 12. Make social connection	1. Education for the users 2. Detection of emergency situation 3. Alert system 4. Social and emotional support 5. Motivation creation 6. Ease of use for elderly 7. Graphical representation of outputs	1. Bio-medical sensors 2. Smart phone 3. PC 4. Motion detector 5. RFID reader	1. Internet 2. Wi-Fi &Wi-Max 3. SMS 4. GSM 5. RFID 6. Zig bee
Hussain A [28]	China	1. Blood pressure M 2. Heart rate M 3. Blood sugar M 4. Oxygen saturation M	1. Central database 2. Information analysis 3. Web-based design 4. Applying web portal	1. Detection of emergency situation 2. Alert system	1. Bio-medical sensors 2. Smart phone 3. PC	1. Internet 2. Wi-Fi &Wi-Max 3. SMS 4. Bluetooth

First author (Reference)	Country/Project	Applications (Usages)	Nonfunctional requirements	Functional requirements	Devices	Communication infrastructures
		5. Respiration M 6. Physical activity M 7. Body temperature M 8. ECG M 9. Galvanic skin response (GSR) M 10. Electromyogram M	5. Applying virtual environment 6. Management of apps 7. Real-time monitoring 8. Intelligent performance 9. Using cloud service 10. Make social connection	3. Social and emotional support 4. Personalized services 5. Graphical representation of outputs 6. Creation user profile	4. Camera 5. Smart wheelchair 6. IoT device	5. GPS 6. Zig bee 7. GSM
Palumbo F [29]	Italy/ GiraffPlus	1. Blood pressure M 2. Heart rate M 3. Weight M 4. Oxygen saturation M 5. Blood sugar M 6. Physical activity M 7. Body temperature M	1. Central database 2. Guideline and standard observation 3. Information analysis 4. Web-based design 5. Applying videoconference 6. Applying virtual environment 7. Management of apps 8. Open and extensible development 9. Real-time monitoring 10. Intelligent performance 11. Applying cloud service 12. System security 13. Make social connection	1. Detection of emergency situation 2. Alert system 3. Display information for the users 4. Ubiquitous information access 5. Personalized services 6. Ease of use for elderly 7. Data visualization ability 8. Graphical representation of outputs 9. Creation user profile	1. Bio-medical sensors 2. Smart phone 3. PC 4. Web-cam 5. Motion detector 6. Camera 7. Apple iPod 8. IoT device	1. Internet 2. Wi-Fi &Wi-Max 3. SMS 4. Bluetooth
Lee J-V [30]	Malaysia/ SEHMS	1. Physical activity M	1. Central database 2. Information analysis 3. Applying virtual environment 4. Real-time monitoring 5. Intelligent performance	1. Detection of emergency situation 2. Alert system 3. Display information for the users 4. Ubiquitous information access 5. Personalized services 6. Ease of use for elderly 7. Graphical representation of outputs	1. Smart phone 2. PC 3. Web-cam 4. Camera	1. Internet 2. Wi-Fi &Wi-Max 3. SMS 4. Bluetooth 5. Phone line

First author (Reference)	Country/Project	Applications (Usages)	Nonfunctional requirements	Functional requirements	Devices	Communication infrastructures
Coradeschi S [31]	Sweden/ GiraffPlus	1. Blood pressure M 2. Heart rate M 3. Weight M 4. Oxygen saturation M 5. Blood sugar M 6. Physical activity M	1. Central database 2. Information analysis 3. Web-based design 4. Applying videoconference 5. Applying virtual environment 6. Management of apps 7. Open and extensible development 8. Real-time monitoring 9. Intelligent performance 10. Android-based 11. Make social connection	1. Detection of emergency situation 2. Alert system 3. Display information for the users 4. Ubiquitous information access 5. Personalized services 6. Ease of use for elderly 7. Data visualization ability 8. Graphical representation of outputs 9. Creation user profile	1. Bio-medical sensors 2. Smart phone 3. PC 4. Web-cam 5. Camera 6. Apple iPod	1. Internet 2. Wi-Fi &Wi-Max 3. SMS 4. Bluetooth
Magaña-Espinoza P [32]	Mexico/WiSPH	1. Physical activity M 2. Heart rate M	1. Central database 2. Information analysis 3. Web-based design 4. Real-time monitoring 5. Intelligent performance 6. Push notification ability 7. System security	1. Detection of emergency situation 2. Alert system 3. Display information for users 4. Ubiquitous information access 5. Data visualization ability 6. Graphical representation of outputs	1. Bio-medical sensors 2. Smart phone 3. PC 4. Motion detector	1. Internet 2. Wi-Fi &Wi-Max 3. GSM 4. Bluetooth 5. 5- LR-WPAN[7]
Saponara S [33]	Italy	1. Blood pressure M 2. Heart rate M 3. Weight M 4. Oxygen saturation M 5. Respiration M 6. ECG M 7. Chest impedance M 8. Medication compliance M	1. Central database 2. Guideline and standard observation 3. Information analysis 4. User-friendliness 5. EPR and PHR development 6. Web-based design 7. Applying audio message	1. Detection of emergency situation 2. Reminder system 3. Alert system 4. Display information for the users 5. Ubiquitous information access 6. Personalized services	1. Bio-medical sensors 2. Smart phone 3. PC	1. Internet 2. Wi-Fi &Wi-Max 3. SMS 4. Bluetooth 5. GSM 6. Zig bee 7. WLAN[8] 8. Ethernet

First author (Reference)	Country/Project	Applications (Usages)	Nonfunctional requirements	Functional requirements	Devices	Communication infrastructures
			8. Open and extensible development 9. Real-time monitoring 10. Intelligent performance 11. Ability to contact HIS[9] 12. Applying SNOMED CT[10] 13. Applying HTTPS[11] 14. System security	7. Graphical representation of outputs 8. Antinational guide 9. Use color for notification		
Ahmed MU [3]	Sweden/ SAAPHO	1. Blood pressure M 2. Heart rate M 3. Weight M 4. Blood sugar M 5. Physical activity M	1. Central database 2. Information analysis 3. User-friendliness 4. Web-based design 5. Real-time monitoring 6. Intelligent performance 7. Applying cloud service 8. System security	1. Reminder system 2. Alert system 3. Display information for the users 4. Ubiquitous information access 5. Graphical representation of outputs 6. Historical summary calculation 7. Recommendation generation 8. Medication management	1. Bio-medical sensors 2. Smart phone 3. PC	1. Internet 2. GSM 3. SMS 4. Bluetooth
de Barros AC [34]	Portugal	1. Physical activity M	1. Applying video linked 2. Applying virtual environment 3. Real-time monitoring 4. Make social connection	1. Education for the users 2. Ubiquitous information access 3. Social and emotional support 4. Motivation creation 5. Personalized services 6. Playing remotely game 7. Ease of use for elderly 8. Use Google TV	1. Smart phone 2. Apple iPod 3. Web-cam 4. Motion detector 5. Camera 6. Game controllers	1. Internet

DOI: http://dx.doi.org/10.5772/intechopen.105568

First author (Reference)	Country/Project	Applications (Usages)	Nonfunctional requirements	Functional requirements	Devices	Communication infrastructures
Tuna G [35]	Turkey	1. Physical activity M 2. Body temperature M 3. ECG monitoring 4. Galvanic skin response (GSR) M	1. Central database 2. Information analysis 3. Real-time monitoring 4. Intelligent performance	1. Display information for the users 2. Ubiquitous information access 3. Graphical representation of outputs	1. Bio-medical sensors 2. Smart phone 3. PC	1. Internet 2. Wi-Fi &Wi-Max 3. SMS 4. Zigbee 5. LR-WPAN
Abo-Zahhad M [36]	Egypt	1. Blood pressure M 2. Oxygen saturation M 3. Respiration M 4. Heart rate M 5. Body temperature M 6. ECG monitoring	1. Central database 2. Information analysis 3. Real-time monitoring 4. Intelligent performance 5. EPR and PHR development 6. User-friendliness 7. Web-based design 8. System security	1. Detection of emergency situation 2. Reminder system 3. Alert system 4. Display information for the users 5. Personalized services 6. Creation user profile	1. Bio-medical sensors 2. Smart phone 3. PC& laptop	1. Internet 2. Wi-Fi &Wi-Max 3. SMS 4. Bluetooth 5. GSM 6. GPRS 7. MMS 8. Cellular network 9. Ethernet
Wannenburg J [37]	South Africa	1. Blood pressure M 2. Oxygen saturation M 3. Heart rate M 4. Body temperature M	1. Central database 2. Information analysis 3. Real-time monitoring 4. Mobile-based design	1. Detection of emergency situation 2. Reminder system 3. Alert system 4. Display information for the users 5. Personalized services	1. Bio-medical sensors 2. Smart phone 3. PC& laptop	1. Internet 2. Wi-Fi &Wi-Max 3. SMS 4. Bluetooth 5. GSM
Ji L [38]	China	1. Blood pressure M 2. Respiration M 3. Heart rate M 4. Physical activity M 5. Body temperature M	1. Central database 2. Information analysis 3. Real-time monitoring 4. Intelligent performance 5. System security	1. Detection of emergency situation 2. Alert system 3. Display information for the users 4. Ubiquitous information access 5. Personalized services	1. Bio-medical sensors 2. Smart phone 3. PC& laptop	1. Internet 2. Wi-Fi &Wi-Max 3. Bluetooth 4. GPRS

First author (Reference)	Country/Project	Applications (Usages)	Nonfunctional requirements	Functional requirements	Devices	Communication infrastructures
Raad MW [39]	Saudi Arabia	1. Blood pressure monitoring 2. Heart rate M 3. Oxygen saturation M 4. ECG M	1. Central database 2. Information analysis 3. Real-time monitoring 4. Intelligent performance 5. User-friendliness 6. System security	1. Detection of emergency situation 2. Alert system 3. Display information for the users 4. Ubiquitous information access 5. Personalized services	1. Bio-medical sensors 2. Smart phone 3. PC& laptop 4. IoT device 5. RFID reader	1. Internet 2. Wi-Fi &Wi-Max 3. SMS 4. RFID 5. Bluetooth 6. GSM

[1]*M* = monitoring.*
[2]*Intel Health Guide is first product in series designed to enable more personalized care management for chronic and age-related disease.*
[3]*Pop-up ads or pop-ups are forms of online advertising on the World Wide Web.*
[4]*Universal Plug and Play (UPP) is a set of networking protocols that permits networked devices, such as personal computers, Wi-Fi access points, and mobile devices to seamlessly discover each other's presence on the network and establish functional network services for data sharing and communications.*
[5]*Radio Frequency Identification.*
[6]*Zigbee is an IEEE 802.15.4-based specification for a suite of high-level communication protocols used to create personal area networks with small, low-power digital radios, such as for home automation, medical device data collection.*
[7]*Low-Rate Wireless Personal Area Network.*
[8]*wireless local area network.*
[9]*HIS: hospital information system.*
[10]*SNOMED CT: Systematized Nomenclature of Medicine Clinical Terms.*
[11]*HTTPS: Hypertext Transfer Protocol Secure.*

Table 1.
Specific extracted data from the given papers.

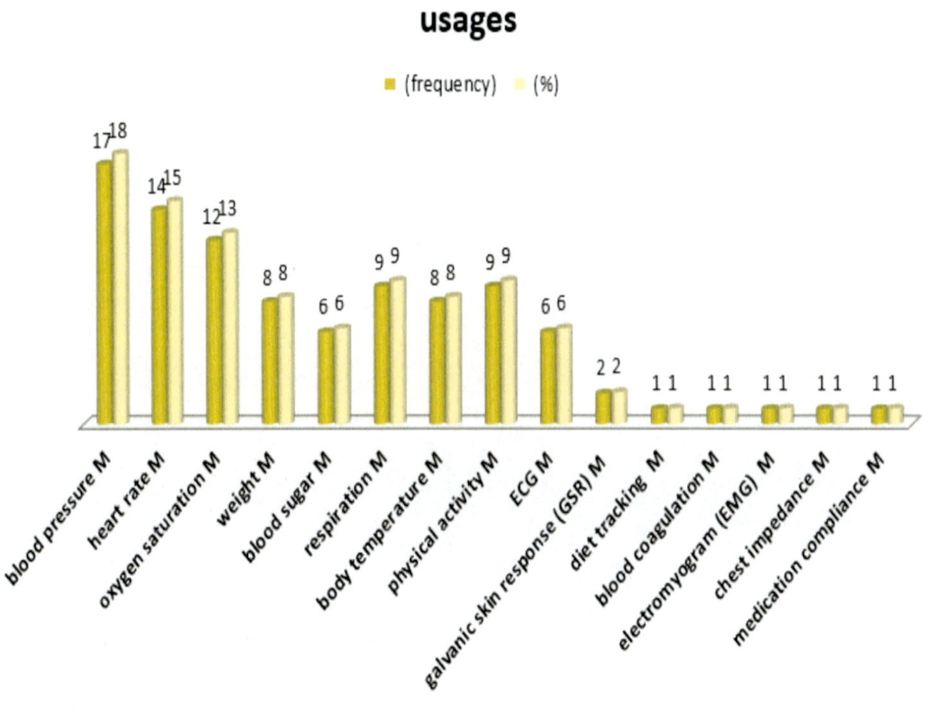

Figure 2.
Frequency and percentage of mostly usages in home telehealth monitoring systems for elderly (M = Monitoring).*

monitoring (15%). The most nonfunctional requirements of these systems included "analysis of information" (12%), and "central database" (11%); the most functional requirements were "display information for the user" and "alert system" (12%), and "personalized services" and "detection of emergency situations" (11%). In addition, results showed that the most commonly used device in the home telehealth systems for the elderly was smart phone (20%) and biomedical sensors (19%); the most widely used communication infrastructure was internet (23%), Bluetooth and Wi-Fi (17%).

Data analysis showed that in recent years (between 2013 and 2019), elderly home telehealth systems have been used by the various countries in the world, mostly in Europe in the form of applied or in progress projects. Furthermore, home telehealth systems for remote monitoring of the elderly living at home were used for a variety of applications. A total of selected articles were analyzed based on 15 parameters. They included blood pressure, heart rate, oxygen saturation, weight, blood sugar, respiration, physical activity, body temperature, electrocardiogram, diet tracking, blood coagulation, galvanic skin response (GSR), electromyogram (EMG), chest impedance, and medication compliance as shown in **Figure 2**.

The functional requirements included "education for the users," "detection of emergency situations," "reminder system," "alert system," "display information for users," "ubiquitous information access," "social and emotional support," "personalized services," "ease of use for elderly," "graphical presentation of outputs," etc. (**Figure 3**).

Nonfunctional requirements included "central database," "information analysis," "user-friendliness," "EPR[2] and PHR[3] development," "web–based design,", "applying

[2] EPR :electronic patient record.

[3] PHR: personal health record.

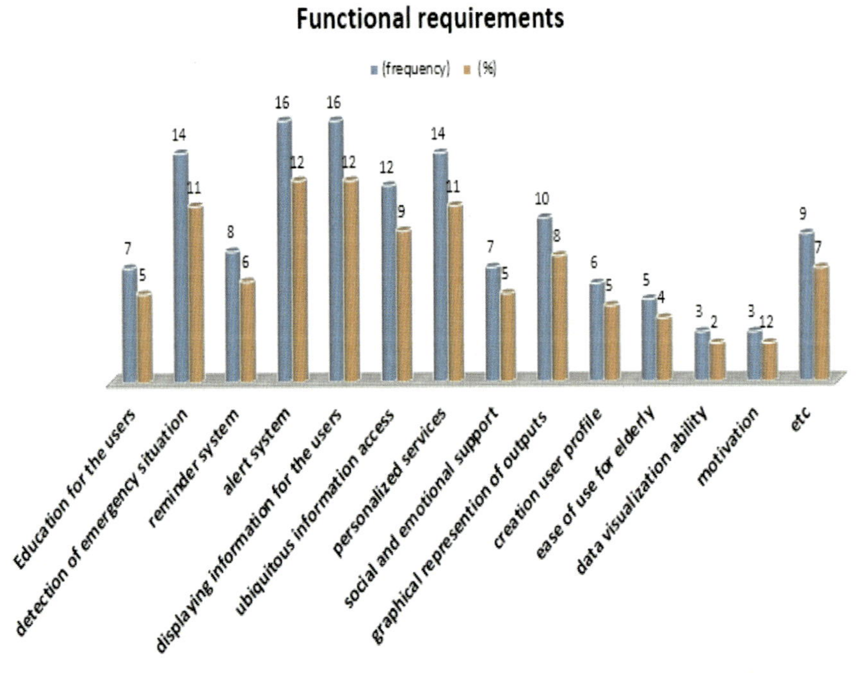

Figure 3.
Frequency and percentage of mostly functional requirements in home telehealth monitoring systems for elderly.

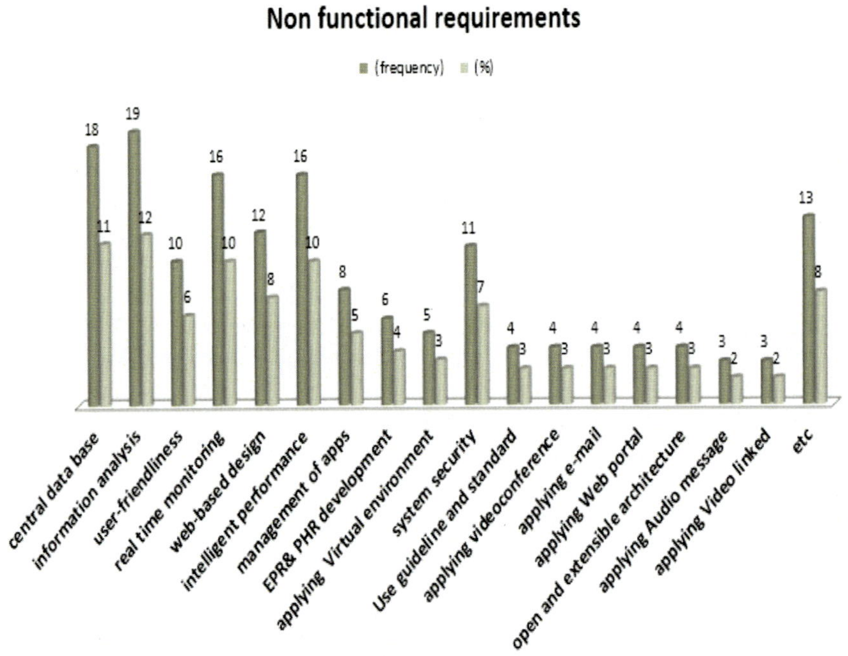

Figure 4.
Frequency and percentage of mostly nonfunctional requirements in home telehealth monitoring systems for elderly etc. including: applying POP – UP (n = 1), service UPnP technology based design (n = 1), animated guide (n = 1), use variety of apps (n = 1), data reduction ability (n = 1), SOCAM & OSGi-based design (n=1), agent-based design (n = 1), applying cloud service (n = 2), push notification ability (n = 1), contact with HIS ability (n = 1), applying SNOMED CT (n = 1), and applying HTTPS (n = 1).*

virtual environment," "management of apps," "creation of user profile," "real-time monitoring," "intelligent performance," "system security," etc. (**Figure 4**).

Different devices were used in elderly health monitoring systems. Seventeen types of devices were mentioned in the articles. They include biomedical sensors, camera, apple iPod, smart phone, PC & laptop, webcam, IoT devices, speaker and microphone, landline phone, pulse-Doppler radar, Intel health guide, broad band router, game controller, activity hub, HTC radar, and X bee PRO S2B module as shown in **Figure 5**.

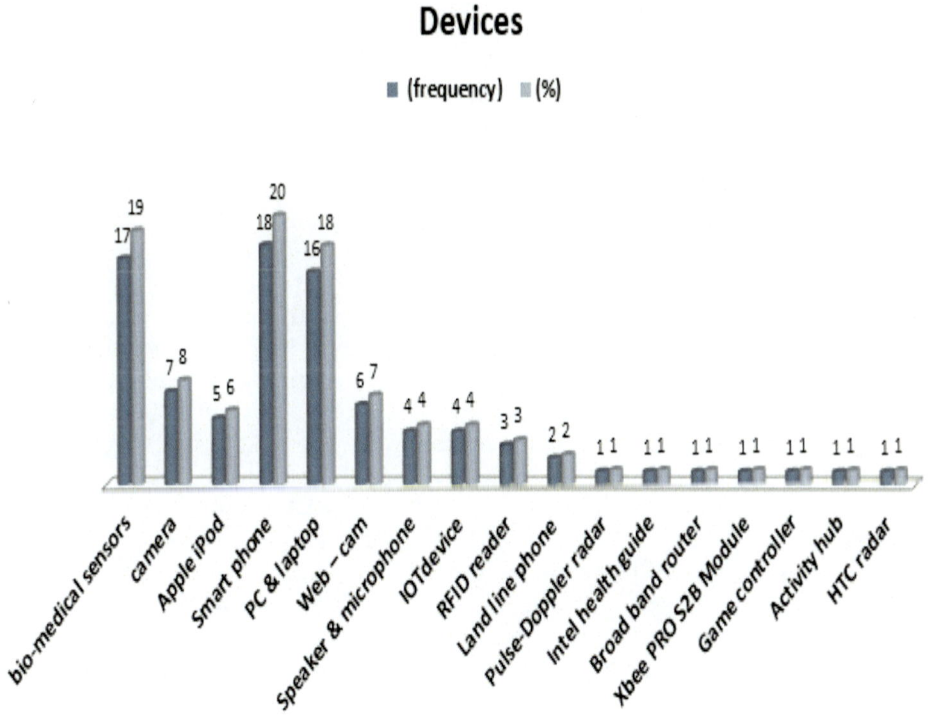

Figure 5.
Frequency and percentage of mostly devices in home telehealth monitoring systems for elderly.

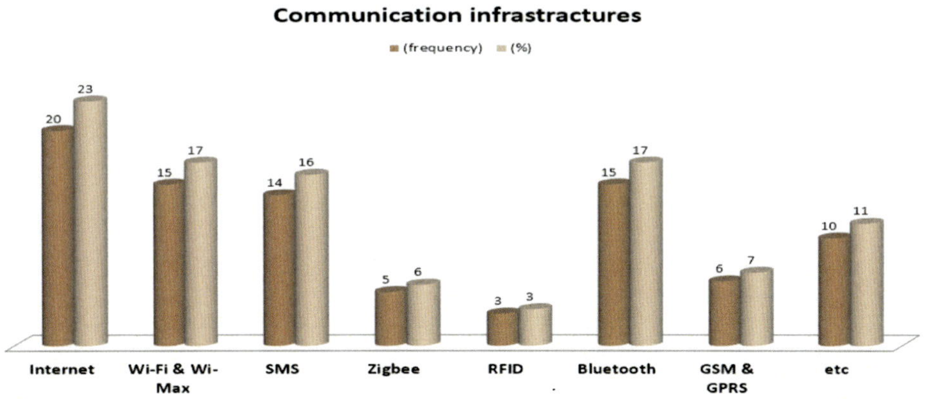

Figure 6.
Frequency and percentage of mostly communications in home telehealth monitoring systems for elderly etc. including: Telephone (n = 2), GPS (n = 1), LR-WPANs (n = 2), WLAN (n = 1), Ethernet (n = 2), MMS (n = 1), Cellular network (n = 1).*

According to the architecture of home telehealth systems, various communication infrastructures were used in these systems such as: Internet, Wi-Fi & Wi-Max, SMS, Zig bee, RFID, GSM & GPRS, and Bluetooth, which are shown in **Figure 6**.

4. Discussion

Home telehealth systems are very much considered, and several large projects are running in various countries. The most abundant applications of elderly remote monitoring system for home telehealth purposes were blood pressure (18%), oxygen saturation (13%), and heart rate (15 %). It is probably due to the importance of examining vital signs for aged people [42]. Hypertension is the most common condition seen in primary care because of its importance; that is, if blood pressure is not timely diagnosed and treated, it might lead to myocardial infarction, kidney failure, stroke, and death [43]. There were various functional requirements that are user-oriented features of home telehealth systems; the most common of them were "display information for the users," "alert systems," "detection of emergency situations," and "personalized services." These functional requirements are extremely important for elderly care due to their responsibility for connecting the user with home telehealth system in order to be utilized practically. According to the fact that aged people may have cognitive impairments, low levels of e-literacy and health knowledge [44], applying functional requirements may support them very much by providing more visual perception and showing the outcomes in the form of understandable graphs and appropriate alerts such as time and dose of medication, observation of nutrition, and daily calorie intakes. Applying home telehealth system may induce data production and collection, which may lead to higher quality of data analysis and results in functions such as detection, prediction, and personalized system outcomes.

The technical features of a software are called nonfunctional requirements [41], They provide infrastructure for the best system interaction with the user (the elderly) and support interoperability and security [45]. They have modules in their structure to meet elderly's needs and support. In this study, the most frequent nonfunctional requirements included "information analysis," "central database," "real-time monitoring," "intelligent performance," "system security," "user-friendliness," and "applying virtual environment." In addition, in home telehealth systems for elderly living at home, various devices and communication infrastructures are used depending on the type of applied telehealth model, architecture, and the distance between home and healthcare center [12]. Based on this review, the most common devices were biomedical sensors and smart phone using Internet, Wi-Fi & Wi-max, and Bluetooth, which are highly frequent ways of communication.

The results of reviewing the projects aimed to monitor elder adults living at home revealed that these systems follow various outcomes such as monitoring purpose systems (sweet-home project) [46] and My Heart[4] [46]. They are aimed to monitor health status in senior people for either telecare or telehealth purposes. For instance, My Heart is a telehealth project to prevent cardiovascular disease by supporting elderly people having proper lifestyle and early diagnosis [47]; REACTION[5] is another

---

[4] MyHeart is a so-called Integrated Project of the European Union aiming to develop intelligent systems for the prevention and monitoring of cardiovascular diseases.

[5] REACTION:Remote Accessibility to Diabetes Management and Therapy in Operational healthcare Networks.

telehealth project to support long-term management of diabetes in elderly cases through using wearable's device, continuous blood glucose monitoring sensors, and automated closed-loop delivery of insulin [48]. However, other well-known elderly monitoring projects are for telecare purposes, they have, particularly in Europe, focused on elderly people's life quality improvement besides extending their independent life through equipping their home and environment [46]. For example, SOPRANO[6] is another project in Europe to develop home environment to support assistive technology using service-oriented architecture (SOA) [49]. InCASA[7] project supports elderly to live longer in their home via increasing their self-confidence [40].

Based on what we learned in this review, the telecare system is composed of telehealth systems which are different, according to the care provided to user. Due to the distinct entity of telecare and telehealth [50, 51], we focused on telehealth as a part of telecare for elderly living at home. Home telehealth system is composed of three parts including elderly home section, service center, and monitoring unit in a healthcare provider center [25, 40]. These three parts are connected to each other and linked to their related devices. The devices are linked too. We focused on one device, which might be a smartphone in elderly's hand; the device encompasses nonfunctional and functional features. Based on the capabilities of a device, different applications would be provided to a user through various communication infrastructures. In fact, the more nonfunctional capabilities are embedded, the more functional features are supported by the device providing more applications for elder adult's remote care at home. Although studied systems are capable of providing various monitoring and care, there is still a need to use new technologies including internet of thing and internet of humans to enhance home telehealth systems. Further research is suggested to proceed this primarily schematic suggestion of home telehealth system for elderly.

5. Limitations

In this study, only requirements and applications of home telehealth systems for elderly living at home were investigated, and further studies are required to examine the effect of these systems on aged people quality of life. Furthermore, in this review, we only focused on home care, and more study might be needed to explore the requirement of telehealth system for nursing home. Another limitation is not studying environmental factors affecting elderly home care and only emphasizing on requirements and applications for health-related factors.

6. Conclusion

Home telehealth systems for monitoring elderly are a type of telemedicine system specifically used for monitoring aged people. They encompass various technologies connected to elderly's home in order to provide different cares. Recognizing all used requirements and achieved capabilities may assist designing more effective systems.

---

[6] SOPRANO: Service-oriented Programmable Smart Environments for Older Europeans.

[7] InCASA: integrated network for completely assisted senior citizen`s anatomy.

They might be expanded in national level to meet elderly's needs in greater scale. Introduced elements of home telehealth system may support developers, nurses, and decision-makers to understand which infrastructure is appropriate for required usages based on available resources and facilities.

Author details

Ahmadreza Shamsabadi[1], Esmaeil Mehraeen[1*] and Zahra Pashaei[3]

1 Department of Health Information Technology, Esfarayen Faculty of Medical Sciences, Esfarayen, Iran

2 Department of Health Information Technology, Khalkhal University of Medical Sciences, Khalkhal, Iran

3 Iranian Research Center for HIV/AIDS, Iranian Institute for Reduction of High Risk Behaviors, Tehran University of Medical Sciences, Tehran, Iran

*Address all correspondence to: es.mehraeen@gmail.com

References

[1] Liu L, Stroulia E, Nikolaidis I, Miguel-Cruz A, Rincon AR. Smart homes and home health monitoring technologies for older adults: A systematic review. International Journal of Medical Informatics. 2016;**91**:44-59

[2] Elledge J. Concordance of motion sensor and clinician-rated fall risk scores in older adults. CIN: Computers, Informatics, Nursing. 2017;**35**(12): 624-629

[3] Ahmed MU, Banaee H, Rafael-Palou X, Loutfi A. Intelligent healthcare services to support health monitoring of elderly. Internet of Things User-centric IoT. 2015:178-186

[4] Chang C-P, Lee T-T, Mills ME. Experience of home telehealth technology in older patients with diabetes. CIN: Computers, Informatics, Nursing. 2017;**35**(10):530-537

[5] Bookey-Bassett S, Markle-Reid M, Mckey CA, Akhtar-Danesh N. Understanding interprofessional collaboration in the context of chronic disease management for older adults living in communities: A concept analysis. Journal of Advanced Nursing. 2017;**73**(1):71-84

[6] Paré G, Jaana M, Sicotte C. Systematic review of home telemonitoring for chronic diseases: The evidence base. Journal of the American Medical Informatics Association. 2007;**14**(3): 269-277

[7] Van den Akker M, Buntinx F, Metsemakers JF, Roos S, Knottnerus JA. Multimorbidity in general practice: Prevalence, incidence, and determinants of co-occurring chronic and recurrent diseases. Journal of Clinical Epidemiology. 1998;**51**(5):367-375

[8] Zhang L, Zeng Y, Fang Y. The effect of health status and living arrangements on long term care models among older Chinese: A cross-sectional study. PloS One. 2017;**12**(9):e0182219

[9] Lee T-t, Huang T-y, Chang C-p, Lin K-c, Tu H-m, Fan C-j, et al. The evaluation of diabetic patients' use of a telehealth program. CIN: Computers, Informatics, Nursing. 2014;**32**(12): 569-577

[10] Spinsante S. Home telehealth in older patients with heart failure–costs, adherence, and outcomes. Smart Homecare Technology and TeleHealth. 2014;**2**:93

[11] Polisena J, Coyle D, Coyle K, McGill S. Home telehealth for chronic disease management: a systematic review and an analysis of economic evaluations. International Journal of Technology Assessment in Health Care. 2009;**25**(3):339-349

[12] Speedie SM, Ferguson AS, Sanders J, Doarn CR. Telehealth: The promise of new care delivery models. Telemedicine and e-Health. 2008;**14**(9):964-967

[13] Arif MJ, El Emary IM, Koutsouris D-D. A review on the technologies and services used in the self-management of health and independent living of elderly. Technology and Health Care. 2014; **22**(5):677-687

[14] Chung J, Demiris G, Thompson HJ. Ethical considerations regarding the use of smart home technologies for older adults: An integrative review. Annual Review of Nursing Research. 2016;**34**(1):155-181

[15] Foster MV, Sethares KA. Facilitators and barriers to the adoption of telehealth

in older adults: An integrative review. CIN: Computers, Informatics, Nursing. 2014;**32**(11):523-533

[16] Ke L-S, Huang X, Hu W-Y, O'Connor M, Lee S. Experiences and perspectives of older people regarding advance care planning: A meta-synthesis of qualitative studies. Palliative Medicine. 2017;**31**(5):394-405

[17] Kim K-i, Gollamudi SS, Steinhubl S. Digital technology to enable aging in place. Experimental Gerontology. 2017; **88**:25-31

[18] Peetoom KK, Lexis MA, Joore M, Dirksen CD, De Witte LP. Literature review on monitoring technologies and their outcomes in independently living elderly people. Disability and Rehabilitation: Assistive Technology. 2015;**10**(4):271-294

[19] Raphael D, Waterworth S, Gott M. Telephone communication between practice nurses and older patients with long term conditions–a systematic review. Journal of Telemedicine and Telecare. 2017;**23**(1):142-148

[20] Madigan E, Schmotzer BJ, Struk CJ, DiCarlo CM, Kikano G, Piña IL, et al. Home health care with telemonitoring improves health status for older adults with heart failure. Home Health Care Services Quarterly. 2013;**32**(1): 57-74

[21] Rantz MJ, Skubic M, Miller SJ, Galambos C, Alexander G, Keller J, et al. Sensor technology to support aging in place. Journal of the American Medical Directors Association. 2013;**14**(6): 386-391

[22] Katalinic O, Young A, Doolan D. Case study: The interact home telehealth project. Journal of Telemedicine and Telecare. 2013;**19**(7):418-424

[23] Dhillon JS, Wünsche B, Lutteroth C. Designing and evaluating a patient-centred health management system for seniors. Journal of Telemedicine and Telecare. 2016;**22**(2):96-104

[24] Vaidehi V, Vardhini M, Yogeshwaran H, Inbasagar G, Bhargavi R, Hemalatha CS. Agent based health monitoring of elderly people in indoor environments using wireless sensor networks. Procedia Computer Science. 2013;**19**:64-71

[25] Lamprinakos G, Asanin S, Broden T, Prestileo A, Fursse J, Papadopoulos KA, et al. An integrated remote monitoring platform towards telehealth and telecare services interoperability. Information Sciences. 2015;**308**:23-37

[26] Chung Y-F, Liu C-H. Design of a wireless sensor network platform for tele-homecare. Sensors. 2013;**13**(12): 17156-17175

[27] Tseng KC, Hsu C-L, Chuang Y-H. Designing an intelligent health monitoring system and exploring user acceptance for the elderly. Journal of Medical Systems. 2013;**37**(6):9967

[28] Hussain A, Wenbi R, da Silva AL, Nadher M, Mudhish M. Health and emergency-care platform for the elderly and disabled people in the Smart City. Journal of Systems and Software. 2015; **110**:253-263

[29] Palumbo F, Ullberg J, Štimec A, Furfari F, Karlsson L, Coradeschi S. Sensor network infrastructure for a home care monitoring system. Sensors. 2014;**14**(3):3833-3860

[30] Lee J-V, Chuah Y-D, Chieng KT. Smart elderly home monitoring system with an android phone. International Journal of Smart Home. 2013;**7**(3):17-32

[31] Coradeschi S, Cesta A, Cortellessa G, Coraci L, Galindo C, Gonzalez J, et al. GiraffPlus: A system for monitoring activities and physiological parameters and promoting social interaction for elderly. In: Human-Computer Systems Interaction: Backgrounds and Applications 3. Springer; 2014. pp. 261-271

[32] Magaña-Espinoza P, Aquino-Santos R, Cárdenas-Benítez N, Aguilar-Velasco J, Buenrostro-Segura C, Edwards-Block A, et al. Wisph: A wireless sensor network-based home care monitoring system. Sensors. 2014;**14**(4): 7096-7119

[33] Saponara S, Donati M, Bacchillone T, Sanchez-Tato I, Carmona C, Fanucci L, et al. Remote monitoring of vital signs in patients with chronic heart failure: Sensor devices and data analysis perspective. In: Sensors Applications Symposium (SAS). University of Brescia, Italy: IEEE; 2012. pp. 553-569

[34] de Barros AC, Leitão R, Ribeiro J. Design and evaluation of a mobile user interface for older adults: Navigation, interaction and visual design recommendations. Procedia Computer Science. 2014;**27**:369-378

[35] Tuna G, Das R, Tuna A. Wireless sensor network-based health monitoring system for the elderly and disabled. International Journal of Computer Networks and Applications (IJCNA). 2015;**2**(6):247-253

[36] Abo-Zahhad M, Ahmed SM, Elnahas O. A wireless emergency telemedicine system for patients monitoring and diagnosis. International Journal of Telemedicine and Applications. 2014;**2014**:4

[37] Wannenburg J, Malekian R. Body sensor network for mobile health monitoring, a diagnosis and anticipating system. IEEE Sensors Journal. 2015; **15**(12):6839-6852

[38] Ji L, Kang T, Tian L, Xiong M, Xiao W, Wu J. Body sensor network for ubiquitous health monitoring. Unmanned Systems. 2015;**3**(02):163-169

[39] Raad MW, Sheltami T, Shakshuki E. Ubiquitous Tele-health system for elderly patients with Alzheimer's. Procedia Computer Science. 2015;**52**: 685-689

[40] Bourque P, Fairley RE. Guide to the Software Engineering Body of Knowledge (SWEBOK (R)): Version 3.0. IEEE Computer Society Press; 2014

[41] Robertson S, Robertson J. Mastering the Requirements Process: Getting Requirements Right. Addison-Wesley; 2012

[42] Kenzaka T, Okayama M, Kuroki S, Fukui M, Yahata S, Hayashi H, et al. Importance of vital signs to the early diagnosis and severity of sepsis: Association between vital signs and sequential organ failure assessment score in patients with sepsis. Internal Medicine. 2012;**51**(8):871-876

[43] Perloff D, Grim C, Flack J, Frohlich ED, Hill M, McDonald M, et al. Human blood pressure determination by sphygmomanometry. Circulation. 1993; **88**(5):2460-2470

[44] Nguyen HT, Kirk JK, Arcury TA, Ip EH, Grzywacz JG, Saldana SJ, et al. Cognitive function is a risk for health literacy in older adults with diabetes. Diabetes Research and Clinical Practice. 2013;**101**(2):141-147

[45] Chung L, do Prado Leite JCS. On non-functional requirements in software

engineering. Conceptual Modeling: Perspective Chapter: Elderly and Telehealth Technology. Springer-Verlag, Berlin Heidelberg: Foundations and Applications; 2009. pp. 363-379. DOI: 10.5772/intechopen.105568

[46] Vacher M, Istrate D, Portet F, Joubert T, Chevalier T, Smidtas S, et al. The sweet-home project: Audio technology in smart homes to improve well-being and reliance. In: Engineering in Medicine and Biology Society, EMBC, 2011 Annual International Conference of the IEEE. Boston, United States: IEEE; 2011. pp. 5291-5294

[47] Habetha J. The MyHeart project-fighting cardiovascular diseases by prevention and early diagnosis. In: Engineering in Medicine and Biology Society, 2006 EMBS'06 28th Annual International Conference of the IEEE. New York: IEEE; 2006

[48] Spanakis EG, Chiarugi F, Kouroubali A, Spat S, Beck P, Asanin S, et al. Diabetes management using modern information and communication technologies and new care models. Interactive Journal of Medical Research. 2012 Oct 4;**1**(2):e2193

[49] Sixsmith A, Meuller S, Lull F, Klein M, Bierhoff I, Delaney S, et al. SOPRANO–an ambient assisted living system for supporting older people at home. In: International Conference on Smart Homes and Health Telematics. Springer; 2009

[50] Fong B, Fong ACM, Li CK. Telemedicine Technologies: Information Technologies in Medicine and Telehealth. New York: John Wiley & Sons; 2011

[51] Stowe S, Harding S. Telecare, telehealth and telemedicine. European Geriatric Medicine. 2010;**1**(3):193-197

Made in the USA
Las Vegas, NV
15 November 2026

c7c75c2b-2002-486d-9209-3a5301b0e89fR05